A Caregiver's Guide to

Alzheimer's Disease

A Caregiver's Guide to
Alzheimer's Disease

300 TIPS
for Making Life Easier

Patricia R. Callone, MA, MRE
Connie Kudlacek, BS
Barbara C. Vasiloff, MA
Janaan Manternach, D Min
Roger A. Brumback, MD

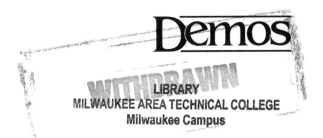

Demos Medical Publishing, LLC
386 Park Avenue South
New York, New York 10016

Visit our website at www.demosmedpub.com

Library of Congress Cataloging-in-Publication Data

A caregiver's guide to Alzheimer's disease :
300 tips for making life easier
/ Patricia R. Callone . . . [et al.]
p. cm.
Includes index.
ISBN 1-932603-16-6 (alk. paper)
1. Alzheimer's disease. 2. Alzheimer's disease—Patients—Care. 3. Caregivers. I. Callone, Patricia R.
RC523.C355 2005
618.97'6831—dc22   2005013869

Made in the United States of America

Contents

Section B – Helpful Information Concerning Alzheimer's Disease or Related Dementia

Section C – Resources Available for Those Affected with Alzheimer's Disease, Their Caregivers, Family Members, and Friends

Preface

Dear Reader,

In 1986 the doctor told me my mother had Alzheimer's disease. I remember standing in the hallway of the doctor's office crying and said, "What am I supposed to do now?"

A lot has happened since 1986, and I have had the opportunity to be a caregiver to three people in my family who had Alzheimer's disease—my mother, my father, and my aunt. I've been either a primary caregiver or secondary caregiver for 18 years. Many people helped me through the long journey of the disease. Their wisdom and compassion contribute to this handbook.

These tips have been put together in a framework to enhance the personal empowerment of all who have Alzheimer's disease as well as their caregivers, family members, and friends.

At each stage of the progression of the disease caregivers, family members, and friends of persons who have Alzheimer's disease or related dementia have two choices: They can concentrate on what capabilities are lost or they can concentrate on what capabilities remain. The choice of where to put the emphasis is crucial for the happiness of persons with the disease, as well as for all those who care for them.

A Caregiver's Guide to Alzheimer's Disease is filled with tips and knowledge that I wish I had had at the beginning of my journey with Alzheimer's disease. Many people have been caring companions, used their expertise, and shared their experiences to help guide me and others to become healthy and competent caregivers. These tips come from persons who live and work on a daily basis with those affected by the disease.

Of special note are these authors and contributors to this book:

CONNIE KUDLACEK has been the Executive Director of the Alzheimer's Association Midlands Chapter for the past 18 years. Caregiving has been a part of Connie's life for over 50 years, beginning when she was very young and caring for her mother, who had cancer. In her mid-thirties, she had the life challenge of caring for her son, who experienced a debilitating head injury at the age of 18. For the past 18 years, she has been involved in program development and the day-to-day management of the Midlands Chapter. She brings a personal as well as professional aspect to her involvement with this book, drawing on her life experiences.

BARBARA VASILOFF is the co-founder of Discipline with Purpose, Inc., a company that features a developmental approach to teaching self-discipline. Barbara has taught for over 25 years; she now works with adults to help them understand the value of self-discipline. When persons are self-disciplined, they have learned to wait and think before acting. This process is important for caregivers who make the journey with a person who has Alzheimer's disease. Because the nature of the disease requires both the person with Alzheimer's disease and the primary caregiver to constantly reevaluate situations, the habit of waiting before acting becomes an invaluable tool for caregivers. Barbara is delighted to contribute her educational expertise to the medical and social service fields to assist persons with Alzheimer's disease.

JANAAN MANTERNACH is co-director of Life, Love, Joy Associates, a company that specializes in writing religious educational and catechetical materials. She also has lectured and conducted workshops throughout the United States and abroad. Caregiving is a new part of her life, because her husband, Carl J. Pfeifer, has been diagnosed with Alzheimer's disease. Although her interest in writing catechetical and educational materials continues, she is finding it necessary to dedicate more of her time to reading and writing about Alzheimer's disease. She feels it is vital to her ongoing personal and professional life to do what she can to help other caregivers, family members, and friends of people with Alzheimer's disease and related dementia.

ROGER A. BRUMBACK is a physician who has been involved with the Alzheimer's Association in different parts of the country. He is presently at the Creighton University Medical Center in Omaha, Nebraska, as Professor of Pathology and Psychiatry and Chairman of the Department of Pathology in the School of Medicine. Here, he provides a medical framework for understanding Alzheimer's disease.

I am vice president for Institutional Relations at Creighton University. I have been a board member of the Alzheimer's Association Midlands Chapter for 6 years and now serve on the Advisory Council. My experience of being both a primary and secondary caregiver to three family members who had Alzheimer's disease has been a wonder-filled journey. Those with the disease have led me down paths that I would never have chosen on my own, and they have helped me in special ways to become a more knowledgeable and compassionate companion to others making their journeys with the disease. I am, indeed, grateful to them. They have inspired me by the unique ways they lived their lives.

Sincerely,
Patricia (Pat) R. Callone

P.S. We would love to hear from those of you who have been diagnosed with Alzheimer's disease, about how you have learned to live with Alzheimer's disease. We would also like to hear from caregivers, family members, and friends of persons with Alzheimer's disease or related dementia. Please pass on the tips that have made life easier for you.

CONTACT: CaringConcepts, Inc., 920 Branding Iron Drive, Elkhorn, NE 68022 or www.caringconcepts.org.

Acknowledgments

We are grateful for the contributions made by the following individuals:

CAROL FEELHAVER, BS, Program Director for the Alzheimer's Association, Midlands Chapter, for your many tips concerning the care of persons with Alzheimer's disease, their caregivers, and families. You have been giving consistent service to persons in Nebraska and Iowa for over 15 years. Your wisdom is found throughout this text.

JEFFREY W. ANDERZHON, AIA, Principal for InVision Architecture, for your contributions concerning the living/built environment for persons with Alzheimer's disease. Your personal experience with your father, who suffered with dementia, and your service on the Board of Directors of the Alzheimer's Association Midlands Chapter, have given us new insights to making pleasant and stimulating living environments for persons with Alzheimer's disease.

VIRGINIA WILLIAMS, BA (deceased), Co-Founder of Care Consultants for the Aging, Inc., and JEFF ALSETH, B.A., President of Care Consultants for the Aging, for the inclusive content found in your *ElderCare Resource Handbook*, Sixth Edition, 2004.

SIOBHAN CHAMP-BLACKWELL, MSLIS, Community Outreach Liaison, and JUDITH R. BERGJORD, M.L.S., Reference Librarian, both from the Creighton University Health Sciences Library, for selecting specific web sites for additional resources that assist persons in many cultures to care for their loved ones.

HELENE LOHMAN, OTD, OTR/L, Associate Professor of Occupational Therapy at the Creighton University School of Pharmacy and Health Professions, for your contributions for understanding and working with the whole person during the progression of Alzheimer's disease.

CAROLYN COFFEY, RSM, Project Manager for Discipline with Purpose, Inc., for your hours of editing the content from twelve contributors.

Introduction

IN OUR FIRST PUBLICATION *Alzheimer's Disease: The Dignity Within: A Handbook for Caregivers, Family, and Friends* (Demos 2006), we focused on the changes that happen in the brain of a person with Alzheimer's disease or related dementia. The purpose of that book was to assist and give support to caregivers who were learning to cope with the personality and behavioral changes occurring in their loved ones. Three different caregiving styles were explained, and the reader had an opportunity to discover his or her own style in working with a person in the Early-to-Mild stage, Moderate stage, or Severe stage of Alzheimer's disease.

The intent of this second book, *A Caregiver's Guide to Alzheimer's Disease*, is to focus on specific tips that will help the person with the disease, and caregivers, family members, and friends to empower the skills, talents, and abilities that remain during the disease progression. You will find tips for persons in all stages of Alzheimer's disease or related dementia. If you have been diagnosed with the disease, you will want to understand what is physically happening in your brain and learn to empower your own special skills and talents throughout the disease progression. Tips for caregivers, family members, and friends also are included, so that they can understand what is physically happening in the brain of a person with Alzheimer's disease. Using this information, caregivers, family members, and friends can help persons with Alzheimer's disease express their desires and help them accomplish what they can throughout the progression of the disease.

In Section A, we divide the progression of the disease into stages: the pre-Alzheimer's stage, when the brain and all its capacities are fully functioning; the early-to-mild stage, which marks the onset of the disease; the moderate stage; and the severe stage. Each chapter starts with a scenario, depicting a daughter and her father going out to eat. These scenarios are intended to help a caregiver understand the changes that can occur because of the progression of the disease. The reader gets a first-hand glimpse of what day-to-day living might be like for the caregiver and the person for whom he or she is caring.

These scenarios are followed by an overview of the specific disease stage and a description of how the disease affects the brain. The circle diagrams found in Chapter I identify the key skills or capacities that are present in the brain: memory, language, complex tasks, social skills, judgment and reasoning, ambulation, and senses. The shaded part of the diagrams shows the brain functions that remain.

General tips for the caregiver are followed by specific tips that will help the person with Alzheimer's disease compensate and cope with the changes that are occurring. These tips are from caregivers and various professionals who, on a daily basis, care for those who have Alzheimer's disease or related dementia. The tips provide the caregiver with ways to focus on the capabilities that remain in spite of losses that might be occurring in the key functions of the brain.

We suggest that you page through the entire book to get an overview of the progression of the disease, and then go back and concentrate on how to use the tips listed for the particular stage in which you find yourself living and working. Be creative about how you make each particular stage as productive as possible for the person with the disease. Because every person is endowed with special talents, skills, and abilities that can be expressed throughout life, look for opportunities to enhance those gifts that remain.

Section B gives the reader insight into the reasons why specific tips have been suggested for the various stages. Frequently asked caregiver questions are answered, and these questions and answers may help caregivers reflect on important issues as they continue in the caregiving process, including:

* Legal and financial issues to consider during the progression of the disease

* Family forums in the caregiving process

* The role of medication and other illnesses in the various stages of the disease

* Helping young children understand what is happening to a loved one

* Handling the holidays and celebrations

* Making the living environment more stimulating and enjoyable

Section C suggests resources, including a listing of Internet resources that can be most useful to gain additional information about the disease and to contact organizations that can be of assistance.

A Caregiver's Guide to Alzheimer's Disease puts information into a framework that helps contribute to the empowerment of the skills and talents of persons with the disease as well as their caregivers, family members, and friends.

A Caregiver's Guide to

Alzheimer's
Disease

Tips for Making Life Easier during the Progression of Alzheimer's Disease

CHAPTER I

Pre-Alzheimer's Stage: Wonder and Worry

Scenario

You and your father have decided to go out to eat at a favorite restaurant, Alexander's Delight. It is his 82nd birthday. You are the person who is closest to your father and live in the same city as he does. Your mother died 3 years ago, and your siblings live in other parts of the country.

"Dad, I'm so glad you chose this restaurant. It is one of my favorites. Are you going to get the chicken-fried steak like you always do?"

"Yes," answers your father. "That just seems right. Your mother and I used to come here often, and she ordered chicken-fried steak too. It was one of our favorites. We had some great conversations over those chicken-fried steak dinners"

Overview of the Pre-Alzheimer's Stage

A PERSON'S BRAIN weighs only about 3 pounds and yet it is the most important part of the body. In a healthy, productive person, all parts of the brain work together to allow the individual access to key brain functions which include:

* Access to long and short term memory

* The ability to utilize language—both verbal and nonverbal

* The ability to complete complex tasks

* The ability and capacity to engage socially with others

* The power of judgment and reasoning

* Use of a full range of bodily movement

* Use of his/her senses to: see, feel, hear, taste, smell, and have the ability to integrate information.

The Key Functions of the Brain in the Pre-Alzheimer's Stage

THE CIRCLE DIAGRAM illustrates the key functions that are controlled by the brain. How well a person is able to do each of

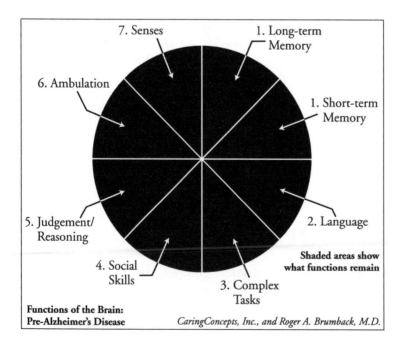

Functions of the Brain:
Pre-Alzheimer's Disease

CaringConcepts, Inc., and Roger A. Brumback, M.D.

these functions is based on innate abilities, education, training and practice, and a person's mental and physical health.

It is the rare individual who has developed each of these functions to the fullest potential. But even the modest ability of a person to perform each of these functions demonstrates that the nerve cells in the brain are healthy and working.

A brief description of the key brain functions follows.

1. Memory in the Pre-Alzheimer's Stage

WHEN A PERSON'S brain is healthy and has been kept active, long-term and short-term memories can be recalled through concentration and focus. Memory cues can help trigger both pleasant and unpleasant memories. These cues include:

* Sight, smell, taste, sound
* Sensations
* People
* Places
* Objects

2. Language in the Pre-Alzheimer's Stage

WHEN A PERSON'S brain is healthy, a person is able to understand sounds and engage in the complex task of communicating effectively with others. Good communicators:

* Recognize and use proper verbal and non-verbal cues. They learn to read the signs of discomfort, stress, frustration as well as pleasure, enjoyment and a sense of well-being in others. They look for a smile or a glint in a person's eye to indicate that communication is effective.

* Are active listeners. They look at the person to whom they are speaking, and they wait for the other person to be attentive before speaking. They will ask the person

questions and repeat back things said to be sure they are understood correctly.

* Avoid sarcasm, slang expressions, or words that would be offensive. They use puns and witty expressions only when individuals they are with enjoy this form of banter.

* Will respect the other person's point of view. They will listen for cues that will let them know how another person or group is feeling.

* Will be positive in outlook, manner, and words.

* Will be gracious and consciously treat persons with dignity and respect.

3. Complex Tasks in the Pre-Alzheimer's Stage

EVERY DAY PRODUCTIVE people can figure out on their own how to accomplish tasks. Useful techniques that help people develop the skills necessary for completing tasks can include:

* Brainstorming about different ways to accomplish a task.

* Selecting the way to accomplish the goal with the best quality and in the given time.

* Making a plan.

* Setting realistic time limits.

* Following through on the plan and making adjustments as changes are needed.

* Evaluating the process and the results to learn from the experience and to improve the ability to complete future tasks.

4. Social Skills in the Pre-Alzheimer's Stage

THE HEALTHY PERSON knows that other people are necessary in life, reaches out to them, and allows others to respond. Social skills remain the glue that keeps people civilized and include:

* Keeping up with personal hygiene and dressing appropriately.

* Interacting appropriately in person, in written communication, via phone or Internet.

* Welcoming the stranger or visitor.

* Acting appropriately and using common courtesies.

* Learning to appreciate diversity.

5. Judgment and Reasoning in the Pre-Alzheimer's Stage

IN THE LATE teenage years, a person's reasoning and judgment become fully formed, and a person is able to do the following:

* Understand and identify problems, often before the problem arises.

* Examine, organize, classify, differentiate, and prioritize.

* Formulate a hypothesis or draw conclusions based on evidence.

* Self-regulate and self-correct.

In short, a person has developed a value system through which his or her world can be filtered.

6. Ambulation in the Pre-Alzheimer's Stage

ACTIVITY AND MOVEMENT are necessary parts of life, and not only keep the person healthy but stimulate the brain. Activities can include:

* Moving from one place to another independently

* Exercising: walking, running, bicycling, swimming, etc.

7. Senses in the Pre-Alzheimer's Stage

PLEASANT SURROUNDINGS can appeal to the senses and enhance the quality of life. These include:

* Appreciating good food
* Sights and sounds of people being with people
* Sharing intimately with others
* Enjoying animals
* Listening to music
* Creating art
* Engaging in spiritual practices

Is It Old Age or Dementia?

FROM TIME TO time in our lives, we can experience a decrease in one or more of the key brain functions. We forget someone's name or momentarily are at a loss for words. We find that it takes us longer to do things that once came so easily. Sometimes these losses can be due to stress, lack of sleep, physical ailments, or even mild depression, and treating these problems can help us get back to normal.

When we observe a continual decrease in key functions of the brain, it is only natural to wonder if it is a sign of old age or if it might indicate that the brain is becoming diseased. The way most people express this concern is to ask the question, "How do I know if I am getting Alzheimer's disease or a related dementia?" or they wonder, "Do I have the beginning stages of Alzheimer's disease or some related dementia?"

The expected changes of aging in the brain have often been called "benign senile forgetfulness," but this is really anything but "benign," since it can cause considerable anxiety in individuals. And this anxiety can actually worsen these symptoms.

What are the things that one can expect as the brain ages? Some of these are rather straightforward (and are really simple lapses in memory):

* Forgetting the name of someone, particularly someone that you have not seen in a while.

* Finding it difficult to recall the right word to express oneself, or even not remembering the name of an object, event, or some other thing, particularly something that is not completely familiar.

One annoying consequence of these changes is that sometimes the individual seems to need prompting to recall the right words.

Things also slow down with age, meaning that it:

* Takes a longer time to learn new skills or grasp new ideas (particularly complicated skills or ideas).

* Takes a longer time to react to things (reflexes slow down, and there is a slowing down in general).

However, a characteristic of the normal aging process is that general intelligence (which medical scientists call "psycho-motor functioning" or "cognitive functioning") remains normal, and reasoning abilities and judgment are not altered.

Symptoms of Alzheimer's disease are actually much more problematic than just the simple lapses in memory, and these symptoms begin to interfere with the ability to perform normal activities. For example:

* Difficulties with ordinary tasks and daily activities—forgetting appointments, directions, or other activities such as: starting the water for a shower and then while leaving the water running getting dressed without taking a shower; problems balancing a checkbook that the individual used to be able to balance; problems with meal preparation or cleanup.

* Making unusual decisions or acting inappropriately.

* Difficulty learning new things—still returning to an old address rather than a new address.

* Dependency—fear of leaving familiar surroundings; suspicious of the activities of others; overly dependent

on others such as familiar family members, but occasionally even strangers.

* Social withdrawal, apathy, and passivity—a loss of interest in activities or friends; tendency to sit watching television or staring into space; sleeping more than usual; speaking and communicating little.

These changes are not sudden, but slowly and progressively become more apparent over many months.

No single behavior can be called characteristic or diagnostic of Alzheimer's disease. However, an individual who has several of these behavioral symptoms likely is experiencing something other than just the normal brain aging process. That something could well be dementia, which is the scientific term used to describe the progressive loss of intellectual abilities as seen in Alzheimer's disease. However, Alzheimer's disease is only one of many brain conditions that can cause dementia. A detailed physical and neurologic examination by a specialist is required to make sure a treatable disorder is not causing the dementia. Once all possible treatable conditions are excluded, it then is likely that the cause of the dementia is a brain disorder such as Alzheimer's disease that is killing nerve cells.

Because people have the ability to self-reflect, the knowledge that something is not right about the way one is functioning causes worry and fear.

* Try to imagine the anxiety when a person thinks, "I don't know why I said or did that."

* Try to imagine what it must be like when a person begins consistently to get lost while driving and can't find his or her way home.

* Try to imagine what it is like to be aware that you can no longer take care of paying bills and other financial matters.

* Try to imagine what it is like to make plans to go out to a show or to dinner, but then consistently forget to show up.

The truth is, if you have been asking yourself over a period of time if something is wrong, you are already aware that it is. You may have been writing yourself notes to help you remember things but now can no longer remember if or why you wrote them. You could even be forgetting to take necessary daily medication. When people do something consistently, and it now affects or interferes with their daily living habits or patterns, they might no longer be dealing with symptoms of aging or benign senile forgetfulness.

> *To the person who cannot remember the past or anticipate the future, the world around her can be strange and frightening.*
> *"Unraveling the Mystery"*—National Institute on Aging

What Is Alzheimer's Disease?

ALZHEIMER'S DISEASE causes the progressive death of nerve cells in the cerebral hemispheres of the brain. The progression of the disease can last for a period of 8 to 20 years, depending on the unique circumstances and health of each person affected. Although there are commonalities, each individual affected with Alzheimer's disease or related dementia experiences the disease uniquely. The disease progresses at its own rate, and the deterioration does not occur in a lock-step, uniform pattern.

For anyone experiencing the onset of the disease—the person affected as well as professionals, caregivers, family members, and friends—there is a period of denial. Many tests are performed to find something else that could be the cause of the behavior changes in the person with the suspected disease. Most of the time, the onset of the disease is very subtle. Only in retrospect does the family put the pieces together and recognize signs indicating the onset of the disease.

It can be frightening to look into the future for persons with Alzheimer's disease, as well as for those who live and work with them. The disease process can last for many years, and yet the person will usually die as a result of something else that is going on in the body at the same time, such as heart disease, cancer, or kidney failure.

When talking about Alzheimer's disease, it is helpful to divide the progression of the disease into stages so that care of individuals can be more easily understood. Although the progression of Alzheimer's disease can be divided into many stages, this book collapses the categorization into just three stages: the Early-to-Mild Stage, the Moderate Stage, and the Severe Stage. (Commonly, researchers have used a division into three, four, or five stages.)

These divisions are like describing the "stages" of a child's growth and behavior—during the child's first year, second year (the terrible two's), teenage years, etc. As the disease progresses the person with Alzheimer's disease gradually loses brain functions and in many ways begins to demonstrate behaviors that are more childlike.

"Staging" of the illness serves the purpose of providing guidelines for making plans for continuous care. This can maximize the person's abilities and preserve his or her dignity. Although there are losses throughout the disease process many skills remain functional.

Because it can be troublesome and even frightening to try to digest all the changes that will occur in the 8–20 year period in which the disease progresses, you may want to read the sections of this book that apply to your needs now. It is best to take one day at a time and be attentive to the needs of the person for whom you are caring.

Even though nerve cells are lost throughout the progression of the disease, some functions remain during all stages. The chart on the following page, prepared by Dr. Roger A. Brumback, shows the progression of the disease and the functions, skills, or capabilities that remain in each stage of the disease.

The Progression of Alzheimer's Disease in the Brain From Roger A. Brumback, MD

What happens in the brain during the Early-to-Mild Stage (generally a 3- to 5-year period)?

* The first area in which nerve cells die as a result of Alzheimer's disease is the memory area of the brain.

A DOCTOR'S PERSPECTIVE: PRESERVED SKILLS

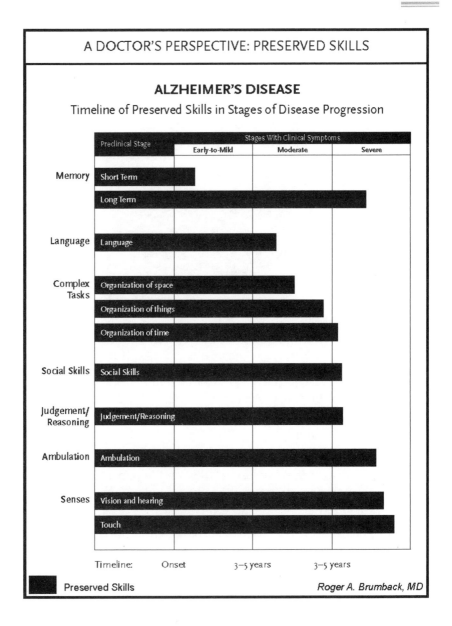

ALZHEIMER'S DISEASE

Timeline of Preserved Skills in Stages of Disease Progression

	Preclinical Stage	Stages With Clinical Symptoms		
		Early-to-Mild	Moderate	Severe
Memory	Short Term			
	Long Term			
Language	Language			
Complex Tasks	Organization of space			
	Organization of things			
	Organization of time			
Social Skills	Social Skills			
Judgement/ Reasoning	Judgement/Reasoning			
Ambulation	Ambulation			
Senses	Vision and hearing			
	Touch			

Timeline: Onset   3–5 years   3–5 years

█ Preserved Skills   *Roger A. Brumback, MD*

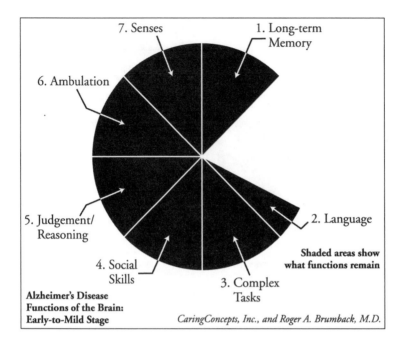

7. Senses

1. Long-term Memory

6. Ambulation

5. Judgement/ Reasoning

4. Social Skills

3. Complex Tasks

2. Language

Shaded areas show what functions remain

Alzheimer's Disease
Functions of the Brain:
Early-to-Mild Stage

CaringConcepts, Inc., and Roger A. Brumback, M.D.

* Because judgment, reasoning, and social skills are still functioning normally, the person can develop compensatory coping strategies to deal with the memory problems.

* Thus, in the beginning stage of the disease process, no one will be aware of the problem because of these compensations and the person will appear normal and often never consult a physician.

What happens as the disease progresses toward the Moderate Stage (generally a 3- to 5-year period)?

* The wave of nerve cell destruction then spreads through the brain. In this stage, the individual has trouble dressing, gets lost or disoriented, and cannot figure out how to use objects.

* This is also the stage of the disease process when driving becomes problematic. The individual cannot integrate all the visual and sound information of the

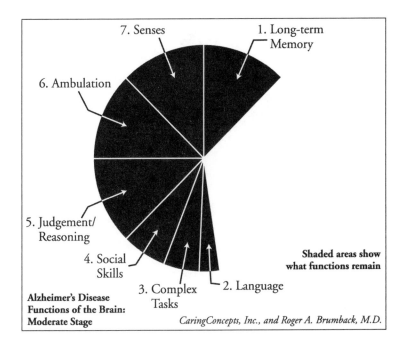

7. Senses

1. Long-term Memory

6. Ambulation

5. Judgement/ Reasoning

4. Social Skills

3. Complex Tasks

2. Language

Shaded areas show what functions remain

Alzheimer's Disease Functions of the Brain: Moderate Stage

CaringConcepts, Inc., and Roger A. Brumback, M.D.

environment with the proper body sensations of the steering wheel and floor pedals.

* This is the time when a person generally consults a physician for an evaluation. Family members and acquaintances become aware that a problem requiring medical evaluation exists.

What happens as the disease progresses into the Severe Stage?

* The person loses the ability to interact properly. This is the stage at which a person often can no longer be managed by caregivers at home. The person loses judgment, reasoning, and social skills.

* Since the median survival (the time by which half the patients die) is 7 years after diagnosis, an individual may die before reaching the Severe Stage of the disease.

* Survival during the Severe Stage depends a lot on the quality of nursing care, since patients lose many of the

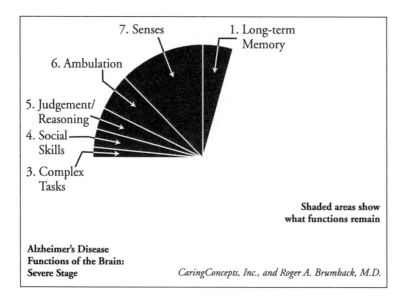

7. Senses

1. Long-term Memory

6. Ambulation

5. Judgement/ Reasoning

4. Social Skills

3. Complex Tasks

Shaded areas show what functions remain

Alzheimer's Disease Functions of the Brain: Severe Stage

CaringConcepts, Inc., and Roger A. Brumback, M.D.

self-care functions that prevent other illnesses. Alzheimer's disease is the underlying cause of death; that is, it weakens the brain's control of body systems and allows other illnesses to end the patient's life.

With knowledge about the disease from the medical chart, the caregiver can translate what is possible—and not possible—to accomplish for the individual with the disease. The second chart, on page 19, was developed by Pat Callone, a caregiver.

A Caregiver's Perspective: Nurture What Remains

Here are some examples of how the information from Dr. Brumback's chart helped me (Pat Callone) understand and care for my father.

What happens during the Early-to-Mild Stage (3 to 5 years)?

Dad was always a very sharp man. He loved to be with people. He had good relationships with his neighbors. He loved candy and gave mints to the children in the neighborhood.

He started having troubles with a neighbor. Dad made a "deal" with a neighbor that if the neighbor would cut his grass all summer, he could have the mower at the end of the summer. Dad didn't remember the "deal" when the neighbor started to take the mower. My husband and I found out about other "deals" he made with the neighbor. We told Dad that we would help him with other arrangements with his neighbor.

What happens during the Moderate Stage (3 to 5 years)?

Dad took his two sisters to the grocery store to do shopping for candy for the children and other items. Instead of backing out of the parking place, he put his foot on the gas and went forward and hit a sign. No one was seriously hurt, and he kept on driving.

On another day, Dad was driving alone and hit two cars. No one was seriously injured. Dad kept saying, "I blanked out. I don't know what happened." We told him the insurance was too high and he couldn't continue driving. He was very unhappy because he had lost his independence.

We found resources from a volunteer organization, and Dad was matched with a lovely woman who came every Thursday to take him to lunch and for a little drive. We found other resources so that someone called or came to his home daily for conversation.

Because Dad was losing the ability to care for himself, he agreed to move to an assisted-living facility with the intention that he would try it out for "a while."

What happens as the disease progresses into the Severe Stage of Alzheimer's?

Dad began to get more serious bladder infections and was having trouble swallowing. Because Dad needed a special diet, he could no longer stay at the assisted-living facility, and he moved to a rehabilitation center and nursing home.

He continued to get many infections that his body could no longer fight. He moved to Hospice House and gradually did not eat. But he did continue sucking on his candy for a while. Finally, he enjoyed a vanilla malt fed to him by means of a syringe. He was at Hospice House about 2 months. His death was very peaceful.

A Life-Altering Experience

OUR LIVES ARE filled with expectations and dreams of promise. Some of those expectations and dreams are fulfilled. Some are not. For persons affected with Alzheimer's disease or related dementia and their caregivers, family members, and friends, life is changed from what was expected.

Respect and love will be present throughout the progression of the disease when caregivers remember that Alzheimer's disease takes away a person's memory but not his mind.

* Respect and love in the Early-to-Mild Stage is shown as a mother tells her caregiving daughter her wishes for medical treatment during the long-term course of Alzheimer's disease.

* Respect and love is shown in the Moderate Stage when persons who have never painted in their life attend Memories in the Making classes—an art project sponsored by local Alzheimer Association chapters—and create the beautiful art works that allow them to express what they are feeling.

* Respect and love is shown in the Severe Stage when, knowing how much her father loved the outdoors, a caregiver pushed his bed out on the patio every sunny day even though her dad could no longer express his wishes with words.

Every person diagnosed with Alzheimer's disease or a related disorder has individual rights throughout all the stages of the disease. Reflecting on these rights can help caregivers adjust their caregiving to recognize the person's dignity throughout the progression of the disease and nurture the functions and capacities that are not lost.

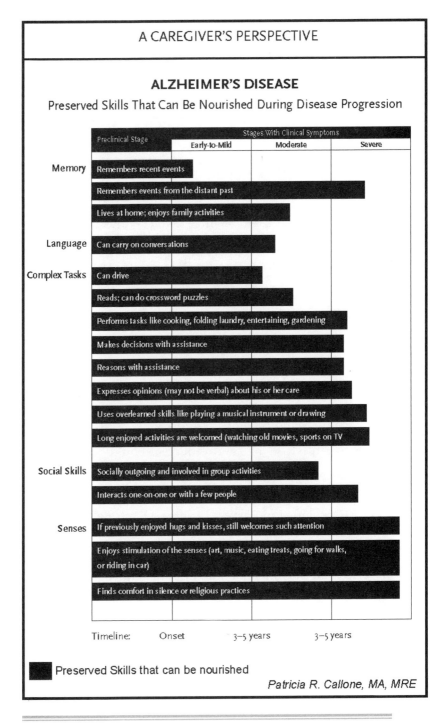

A CAREGIVER'S PERSPECTIVE

ALZHEIMER'S DISEASE
Preserved Skills That Can Be Nourished During Disease Progression

	Preclinical Stage	Stages With Clinical Symptoms		
		Early-to-Mild	Moderate	Severe
Memory	Remembers recent events			
	Remembers events from the distant past			
	Lives at home; enjoys family activities			
Language	Can carry on conversations			
Complex Tasks	Can drive			
	Reads; can do crossword puzzles			
	Performs tasks like cooking, folding laundry, entertaining, gardening			
	Makes decisions with assistance			
	Reasons with assistance			
	Expresses opinions (may not be verbal) about his or her care			
	Uses overlearned skills like playing a musical instrument or drawing			
	Long enjoyed activities are welcomed (watching old movies, sports on TV			
Social Skills	Socially outgoing and involved in group activities			
	Interacts one-on-one or with a few people			
Senses	If previously enjoyed hugs and kisses, still welcomes such attention			
	Enjoys stimulation of the senses (art, music, eating treats, going for walks, or riding in car)			
	Finds comfort in silence or religious practices			
Timeline:	Onset	3–5 years	3–5 years	

■ Preserved Skills that can be nourished

Patricia R. Callone, MA, MRE

Patient's Bill of Rights

* to be informed of one's diagnosis

* to have appropriate, ongoing medical care

* to be productive in work and play as long as possible

* to make care decisions for him/herself when he/she can

* to choose the medical treatment he/she wants

* to be treated like an adult, not like a child

* to have expressed feelings taken seriously

* to be free from psychotropic medication if at all possible

* to live in a safe, structured, and predictable environment

* to enjoy meaningful activities to fill each day

* to be out-of-doors on a regular basis

* to have physical contact including hugging, caressing, and hand-holding

* to be with persons who know one's life story, including cultural and religious traditions

* to direct how his/her resources should be used

* to be cared for by individuals well-trained in dementia care.

(Developed in part by Virginia March Bell, MSW and David Troxel, MPH)

Through the use of charts, diagrams, scenarios, and tips we offer you our understanding of Alzheimer's disease and hope you find some ways to make your life easier and happier through the fulfillment of new dreams and new expectations.

CHAPTER II

Early-to-Mild Stage: Something's Going Wrong

Scenario

You and your father have decided to go out to
eat at a favorite restaurant, Alexander's Delight. It
is his 85th birthday. When you walk in, your dad
says, "This is a nice place. Look at the plates on
the wall and the Fifties' decorations. Your mother
would have loved this." You are surprised and say,
"Dad, we've been here a hundred times before.
Don't you remember?" "No we haven't," he re-
sponds. "This is the first time for me." You let the
conversation move on to other things. It is time to
order from the menu. Your dad says, "I think I'll
have the chicken-fried steak. That sounds good."
You respond, "Yes, I'll have our favorite dinner
together. You and mom used to like that dinner,
too." Your dad says, "What do you mean? My
favorite dinner is spaghetti and meatballs." You
say, "Dad, when we were here on your 82nd birthday, you said that you and Mom used to come
here all the time . . . and that you liked chicken-
fried steak." Your dad begins to answer back and
argue. The dinner was not as pleasant as when you
were celebrating his 82nd birthday.

Overview of the Early-to-Mild Stage

WHEN THE WORRY AND WONDER HAVE CEASED, and the diagnosis has been made that your loved one has Alzheimer's disease, you will find yourself moving from being a temporary caregiver to the realization that your caregiving will now be permanent. Looking over the past few months or years, you probably can identify many signs that were present pointing to this day. This is the time to seriously learn as much as you can about the changes that will occur in the brain and will eventually affect each of the key skills and capacities that we often take for granted when things are going well.

This is the time to develop a new mindset regarding Alzheimer's disease. While you may be anxious because of the losses you experience in your loved one, you can choose to focus on these losses and perhaps become overwhelmed, or you can begin to look for the positive signs of life and dignity that remain. Instead of wishing that your life would unfold the way you always pictured it would, you can embrace what is happening and realize this is your life now. It can be as equally fulfilling if you slowly change the way you think about life's circumstances, letting go of some things and embracing others.

This new mindset requires us to think about ourselves and the adjustments we have to make to cope with the disease. We need to think more creatively about finding ways to help the person with Alzheimer's disease compensate and feel empowered.

Because of prevalent attitudes about aging and dementia that exist in contemporary society, it is easy to forget or fail to acknowledge that persons with Alzheimer's disease still have the capacity to self-reflect and the desire to be contributing members of society. When we fail to change the way we think about Alzheimer's disease, we run the risk of acting inappropriately or unintentionally hurting our loved ones.

It helps to remember that not all the key brain functions will diminish at the same time, and much remains. When we forget or fail to acknowledge the remaining functions, negative actions can become part of our caregiving style. We may:

* Speak to persons with Alzheimer's disease as if they were a child or simply ignore them when memory fades.

* Laugh at their attempts to communicate, or stop trying to figure out what they want to say as language diminishes.

* Do things for them or refrain from asking them to do things for themselves when they can still complete some complex task.

* Be reluctant to bring them to family gatherings, as social skills diminish.

* Be embarrassed over their actions when reasoning and judgment become faulty.

* Avoid taking them into public, as walking becomes more labored.

* Forget or fail to create a stimulating and aesthetically pleasing environment, as their senses are affected, because we don't think they are capable of enjoying their surroundings.

When we look for the dignity within persons who have Alzheimer's disease, we look for ways to help them compensate, cope, and adapt to their ever-changing lifestyle. We remember that the ability to self-reflect will continue despite the disease. Finding ways to empower persons to continue to be productive and of value in life will be part of our new mindset. We might:

* Find pictures and ask them questions about what they remember about the pictures to help trigger their long-term memory when short-term memory fades.

* Play games, such as having them identify objects around the house to stimulate language as long as possible and converse with them in their native language.

* Think about activities they learned before the brain became diseased, and set aside time for them to still do these activities, such as painting, taking pictures,

gardening, or other hobbies. The ability to perform complex tasks that have been learned early often will remain throughout the course of the disease.

* Invite people to call on the phone on a regular basis, or take walks or set the routine to visit a local restaurant to keep socializing.

* Accept the fact that inconsistencies exist in reasoning and judgment and know that we will have to make decisions to keep them safe.

* Find safe places to walk or take drives in the car and play games to stimulate movement.

* Play music, continue to decorate the house for holidays, or simply set a nice table to provide a stimulating environment that will appeal to the senses.

Everyone wants to be treated with dignity and respect. Here are some examples of persons with the disease and their self-reflection about the disease itself:

* A clinical nurse with Alzheimer's disease shared: "I've lost my memory but not my mind. Because of my profession I can reflect on myself as a 'patient' and see what is happening sometimes."

* A business man who used to work in a Fortune 500 company stated: "I used to manage many things. I still want to do what I can do. Please don't give me envelopes to lick and think that fulfills me."

* A mother used to sew all the clothes for her family, including men's suits, hats, and the like. When given some needlepoint to do with her daughter, she tried to do it, looked at the daughter, and with disgust threw the materials on the floor.

* A husband said to his wife: "Do I still have my mind? I must have been very bad in my life to have God give me this. My life isn't supposed to be this way."

* A former professor at a university reflected: "I don't understand why they won't let me go to church alone.

It is just across the street. I used to teach in foreign countries. I know how to get places."

* A wife caring for her husband who has Alzheimer's disease remarked: "Throughout our marriage, we said to each other daily, 'I love you!' These were never empty words, even when we were angry with one another. We continue to do that today, except we seem to do it more often. Most of the time, in the past, I was the initiator in these daily affirmations of affection. Today, he initiates them more, and I find healing in the truth that he continues to consciously and actively love me." (From *Alzheimer's Disease: The Dignity Within: A Handbook for Caregivers, Family, and Friends.*)

Changes in the Brain in the Early-to-Mild Stage

ALZHEIMER'S DISEASE CAUSES the slow, progressive death of nerve cells in the cerebral hemispheres of the brain. The brain is different from other organs of the body in that every nerve cell in the brain does something unique that only that nerve cell can do and no other nerve cell can do. In the brain, every part has a specific function, and all the parts must work together for the brain to work correctly. Loss of any part of the brain results in loss of that function, because no other part of the brain can take over or perform that function.

The first area in which nerve cells die in Alzheimer's disease is located near the center of the cerebral hemispheres: the hippocampus. The hippocampus is the memory area of the brain. All memory is cataloged and recorded by the hippocampus.

As Alzheimer's disease progressively consumes brain functions, those that remain must be cherished and, with caregiver's assistance, displayed more prominently.

The first symptom noticeable in the Early-to-Mild stage of Alzheimer's disease is memory loss. The rest of the brain works normally, however, so the person still moves, and feels things, sees, hears, and integrates information. Because judgment, reasoning, and social skills are still normal, the person can develop compensatory coping strategies to deal with the memory problems.

Thus, in this beginning stage of the disease process, probably no one will be aware of the problem; because of these compensations, the person will appear normal and never consult a physician. As Alzheimer's disease progresses, the damage to the brain moves from the hippocampus to the temporal lobe, causing the person to have trouble understanding words or expressing the correct words. Difficulty using or understanding words can cause conflicts with others and also cause the individual to withdraw and communicate less. Because the frontal lobes are still intact, the person tries to understand why others do not seem to respond appropriately to conversation.

The focus during this Early-to-Mild stage should be on the abilities, skills, and talents that remain and can be used and nourished. Instead of worrying about losses, concentrate on nourishing the remaining skills and abilities.

Tips to Assist the Caregiver in the Early-to-Mild Stage

WHEN YOU BECOME a caregiver to someone in the Early-to-Mild stage of Alzheimer's disease, the first thing you might notice is a struggle between wanting to do things for the person who has been diagnosed and wondering if you should. You might wonder, "Is it better to allow persons to be independent and do things for themselves (although sometimes in a different way) or to rescue them and do things for them?"

In the Early-to-Mild stage of Alzheimer's disease, a caregiver will find it most productive to refrain from doing things for persons that they can do for themselves and to encourage independence as much as possible. The caregiver's task is to act as an advocate and resource person. Observe without interfering, unless an activity involves potential physical danger or abuse. Think about the times when it would be best for you to let the person with Alzheimer's disease take control, when you should share decision-making powers, and when you should take the lead. In addition:

✳ Learn as much about the disease as you can, before problems arise. Be proactive.

✳ Go to your family physician for a thorough medical exam when you suspect something is wrong, and visit a geriatric assessment center or other medical facility specializing in Alzheimer's disease or dementia. Many things can cause dementia, and sometimes the dementia can be helped, although often it is irreversible.

✳ Try to understand and talk about the brain functions that remain and those that are lost, based on what the person with dementia is experiencing.

✳ Share with others in the family who want to know more about the disease any and all information that you have.

✳ Call a family forum to discuss life transitions as well as changing stresses in the family. Consider including the person with dementia in this discussion.

✳ Be ready for your own denial, and denial by your loved one and other family members, that the disease is affecting someone you care deeply about.

✳ Be open in discussing with others the information that you, your spouse, or a friend has Alzheimer's disease.

✳ Talk with a spiritual counselor about your feelings. A counselor can help sort out what is fact and what is feeling.

✳ Seek counsel with your relatives, friends, and counselors at the local chapter of the Alzheimer's Association. If you are your own caregiver, lay out a plan for your long-term comfort and care.

✳ Identify family, friends, and outside sources who will assist you when you carry the burden of full responsibility for overseeing all issues of daily life.

✳ Be prepared to take the leadership role in all activities of daily living: It is important that all financial and legal documents be put in place while the person with Alzheimer's disease can be a part of that process.

* Educate yourself on the resources available from the local or national chapters of the Alzheimer's Association. Even a limited knowledge can help you help others you meet who might become a caregiver to a person with Alzheimer's disease or related dementias.

* Review the charts in Chapter I of this book as you anticipate the new challenges that will come with the progression of the disease. Also, consult the Alzheimer's Association local chapter, which has materials for you to learn about the subtle changes that arise in each of the key functions of the brain as the disease progresses.

* Be an active listener and really hear what is important to the person for whom you are caring. He may want to talk about sensitive issues such as long-term care or power of attorney. He may want to tell you things he is aware of that are causing him concern. Remember that the disease will set the pace for what is to come. In many cases, the person for whom you are caring may not want to prepare for the future. Don't force this kind of dialogue; simply move forward on these issues at his pace. Sometimes, too, your physician will suggest that certain steps must be taken. Follow them when you can.

Having Alzheimer's disease or being a caregiver often causes one to ask questions such as: "What is my purpose in life? What am I supposed to do now? How am I to live life in the most productive way possible?"

For the caregiver, it is a matter of keeping in mind the dignity within the person who has the disease and constantly finding ways to honor that dignity. Help the person grow and mature with the capabilities that she still has. Try to have enough self-discipline to stop before you speak or act and think "What is going on here? Is the person for whom I am caring really intentionally doing this or that . . . or saying this or that ... to make life difficult, or is it the disease acting out instead?"

For the person with the disease, it is a matter of continuing to do what is possible, as long as possible. Find ways to cope with situations that will help you remember current appointments, people who have called, and other details of daily life. Throughout life, everyone has to deal with losses ... whether caused by Alzheimer's disease or not.

1. Memory in the Early-to-Mild Stage

MOST CAREGIVERS OF PERSONS with Alzheimer's disease know clearly that the disease will first impact a person's short-term memory. Something important for the caregiver to remember is that persons with Alzheimer's disease generally also know they are losing their memory. If possible, early in the disease process, identify those things that are really important. Then utilize the following tips to help a person realize what she wants out of life. Keeping dignity in your relationship includes being able to distinguish and accept what an individual wants and what she truly needs to feel whole. Activities that are habitual will still be possible and can help the person with dementia feel productive.

Set up memory clues:

* Make lists, use pictures, outline simple steps, keep routines consistent.

* The loss of short-term memory will mean the person needs prompting and cues to know what to do.

* Keep duplicate house and car keys. Find an obvious place to hang them, so that they will be easy to find in the event the person with Alzheimer's disease forgets where the keys were put. At the same time, you must reevaluate whether driving should be permitted.

* Mark where items are stored in the kitchen and bathroom. Place labels on drawers, cupboards, and the

dressers. Use calendars, pill boxes, and other memory aides.

* Frame questions and instructions in a positive way. Know that the person is usually aware of a loss of skills and can become frustrated with his increasing dependence on others.

2. Language in the Early-to-Mild Stage

LANGUAGE BEGINS TO deteriorate in the Early-to-Mild stage, so that conversations with a person with Alzheimer's may become more difficult. Finding the right words to fully express what she is feeling can be problematic. As a caregiver, continue to act as a resource, and help the person express herself. If the person with Alzheimer's disease finds it humorous when she cannot find the correct word and can laugh with the caregiver when the word is finally found, enjoy the humor. If appropriate, provide a missing name or word so that the person does not get frustrated.

Coach and cue:

* Set the mood for interactions with the person with dementia. Try a calm, gentle, matter-of-fact approach. Your relaxed manner can be contagious.

* Look directly at the person and make sure you have her attention before you begin to speak. If you cannot get the person's attention, wait a few minutes and try again.

* Talk in positive terms. Limit the number of "don'ts" and avoid giving harsh or direct orders.

* Try not to finish sentences for persons with dementia. This can be embarrassing for them. Give them time to communicate and find the appropriate words, but if and when the appropriate words are not forthcoming, gently suggest what the person might want to say. Often the person with Alzheimer's disease will look to

you for help. Try to help before the person gives up in frustration.

* Speak slowly, repeat what you said if necessary, using different words or short sentences. Ask for feedback, and look for feedback in body language and facial expressions.

* Try never to use a condescending tone of voice when you are speaking slowly and in short sentences, because a condescending tone can provoke anger. It is difficult to be patient when communicating in this manner. Remember that communicating properly reveals respect and helps maintain the person's dignity. However, when you've "lost it," a sincere apology will demonstrate your respect.

* Ask simple questions that require the choice of a "yes" or "no" answer, rather than open-ended questions. Instead of saying, "What would you like to wear today?" you could ask, "Do you want to wear this green shirt or this red one?" or "This dress looks so good on you, how about wearing it today?" An interest in the choice of clothing may remain long after the person can't choose for himself, so keep him informed with words like, "This is what you'll wear tomorrow." Or, "This will be a perfect outfit for what we're doing tomorrow."

* Don't treat the person with Alzheimer's disease as non-existent when you are communicating in a group. Let the person with the disease respond, and don't answer for him. This is especially important at medical appointments, where you must help him maintain dignity by not answering for him.

Express your feelings:

* Don't be afraid to share your feelings with persons who have Alzheimer's disease. It lets them know that you still need them and value their thoughts and opinions.

* Express your feelings to help you release tension and help comfort the person. This is especially important

after you have been really angry and frustrated and have "lost it" with him.

* Be positive, optimistic, and reassuring to the person. Use such expressions as "Everything will be OK." "Don't worry." "We're doing great." "We're going to see this through." "I'm here to help you."

* Avoid discouraging the person from talking about difficult and emotional subjects such as dying. Don't reject or dismiss feelings with statements like "That's not going to happen."

* Use the person's name, instead of referring to the person with Alzheimer's disease as "he" or "she."

3. Complex Tasks in the Early-to-Mild Stage

IN THE EARLY-TO-MILD stage, persons can still drive, enjoy reading, and enjoy doing crossword puzzles and games. They can perform tasks such as cooking, folding laundry, gardening, and entertaining. They can still make decisions (sometimes with assistance), and they can still reason and show good judgment.

A person with a dementing illness depends on a certain amount of structure in daily routines. This consistency is important in helping to minimize the amount of stress the person with memory loss experiences. Multistep tasks that might have been readily performed in the past now need to be broken into separate individual tasks. Tasks done frequently and repeatedly before Alzheimer's disease are often retained the longest. In addition, consider the following tips.

Structure situations for success:

* Be aware of the amount of time the person with Alzheimer's disease can attend to a task. Look for signs that frustration is beginning to set in, and divert his attention before the stress becomes overwhelming.

* Do not rush in to help a person with Alzheimer's disease when he is struggling with dressing, putting

clothes back in a closet, opening a car door, setting the table, and other relatively simple activities. Most times, he will accomplish the task if allowed to keep working at it. Only when he asks for help should you intervene. Accept the fact that a task may not be as carefully done as it might have been before the onset of Alzheimer's disease.

* Avoid taking responsibilities away from the person through such comments as, "Here! You can't do that. Give it to me." Instead of assuming that the person can't do certain tasks, put the emphasis on what the person can perform. Sorting coins or stacking papers, unloading the dishwasher, and working with a care-giver on repetitive activities can be very satisfying.

* Coordinate all clothing into sets to help eliminate confusion about what to wear. This allows the person with dementia to choose appropriately and to remain some-what independent.

* Try to be generous when the person wants to help; let him help you. Keep adjusting the task so that he feels useful.

* Work side-by-side with the person, particularly on tasks he may have difficulty accomplishing alone. This can be a real challenge at times, because doing a task together could take twice as long and demand more patience than you have.

* Set routine times for eating, playing games, socializing, and quiet reflection.

* Have a schedule of daily activities posted in an easily accessible place as a reminder of what is to take place that day or what will need to be accomplished.

* Provide the person with Alzheimer's disease with a large monthly calendar to keep track of appointments, trips, and special occasions. Some persons become anxious about upcoming events and frequently ask when they will happen. Circle events in bold coloring and

mark each passing day with an X to help them deal with the concept of time.

* Use medication holders with timers to signal when medicine is due. Or get into a habit of dispensing the medicines at the same time every day. If you're going to be out together during one of the times, carry the doses with you in small medicine cases. Dispensing the medicine can be done discreetly and easily.

* Remain as flexible as possible to accommodate the changing moods of the person with dementia. Rigid schedules should be avoided.

* Look for ways to adjust the environment to accommodate the person's changing needs.

* Use soap on a rope to eliminate the possibility that the person could slip and fall on the soap while in the shower or tub.

* Purchase those appliances, such as electric coffee makers, teapots, and irons, that turn off automatically after a short period of time.

4. Social Skills in the Early-to-Mild Stage

AS YOUR TASK OF being a caregiver to a person with Alzheimer's disease or other dementia grows, you must determine if the person with Alzheimer's disease had a familiar custom or traditional way of doing things. Ask yourself: "Can I honor that custom, or do I need to modify it?" and "If I were in this position, what would I like someone to do for me?"

In the Early-to-Mild stage, the person could still be very outgoing and involved in group activities. The person may enjoy interacting one-on-one or with a few people at the same time. Ask yourself what will make the person comfortable. What is she able to handle? What will make her happy? If the person had excellent social skills before the disease, and this was a strong part of her personality, it can remain. In addition, consider the following tips.

Respect and accommodate the need for socialization:

* Arrange for a senior companion or a friend to visit weekly, to take the person with Alzheimer's disease to the movies or zoo or to shop.

* Keep including the persons with Alzheimer's disease in those social events that were part of their lives before the illness occurred. This can sometimes be hard, because of the effort it requires. However, mingling with others enriches the spirit, can be a relief, and can provide unexpected moments of pleasure.

* Be aware that persons with Alzheimer's disease become more dependent on the primary caregiver and can become agitated when that person is not within sight. The person with Alzheimer's disease may often "shadow" the caregiver, thus preventing the caregiver from experiencing any private time.

* Set up some parameters for privacy, alone time, or quiet times, such as when you're working on your computer, preparing a meal, or reading a book. These private times, if gently but firmly protected, will often be respected by the person with Alzheimer's disease.

* Remember that keeping up personal hygiene and dressing appropriately, while extremely important to the fully functioning adult, will often gradually become less important in the life of the person with Alzheimer's disease. However, sometimes it can remain important even when he needs more and more assistance with all aspects of personal care. Being well groomed and well dressed adds to a person's dignity, self-respect, and well-being. It also provides a sense of well-being to the caregiver.

* Keep your sense of humor and be willing to share laughter.

5. Judgment/Reasoning in the Early-to-Mild Stage

WHEN PERSONS ARE in the Early-to-Mild stage of Alzheimer's disease, the caregiver can be an observer, watching closely that the loved one is safe in her independent choices.

Keep 'em sharp:

* Remember that early in the disease process, the person with Alzheimer's disease can participate in setting up legal and financial documents to take care of future needs. Many times, persons with Alzheimer's disease will come to terms with the fact that they have the disease and will want to arrange for future long-term care.

* Monitor yourself to make sure that, as caregiver, you are not in denial and placing roadblocks. Assist persons with Alzheimer's disease to complete necessary documents, and do not deny them the opportunity to do so when they are ready.

* Be open to questions or discussions regarding why things are changing. As the person moves out of denial, he may ask, "Why is this happening to me?"

* Help the person with Alzheimer's disease to self-reflect on what is easy or difficult for her to do.

* Help the person with Alzheimer's disease label emotions by making such comments as: "You look sad." "Is this frustrating for you?" "You are feeling angry right now. You know it is OK to feel angry."

* Try to understand why certain difficult behaviors are occurring. What are some of the factors triggering the behavior? What are the factors that you can change? It is important to try to recognize elements in the environment, the medical situation, or problems related to communication that are contributing to the problem.

* Keep a daily log or a record describing problems or challenges. Jot down the time and what happened in as much detail as possible. Think about what was going

on right before the behavior occurred. Who was involved? Who was affected by the behavior? What emotion was expressed by the confused person? Anger? Frustration? Fear? Did the caregiver's approach resolve the situation? Did that approach fail or end in frustrating or irrational behavior? This log can be helpful in identifying patterns in frustrating behaviors.

* Have regular vision and hearing check-ups to help the person with Alzheimer's disease maintain his abilities as long as possible or compensate for declines. Impaired vision or hearing are two problems that can affect a person's ability to understand.

6. Ambulation in the Early-to-Mild Stage

THE PERSON IN THE Early-to-Mild stage of Alzheimer's disease generally has full use of movement. Allow the person to enjoy independence as long as possible. Encourage exercise and safe ambulation.

Keep 'em active:

* Be aware that problems with ambulation show up slowly, and come and go depending upon the circumstances. For example: While waiting in line, taking a few steps forward and then stopping can become confusing. You may have to gently keep urging the person forward. Avoid walking on shiny surfaces, as these surfaces can appear icy or slick to persons with dementia.

* Leaving a crowded place can also be a challenge, because the person with Alzheimer's disease may become frightened by all the movement and want to hold back.

* Getting out of cars can take longer, and walking into a store or other building can become slower. Telling a person with Alzheimer's disease to "hurry up" doesn't help. It's important to be aware that the person has fallen behind you and that you need to slow your pace.

* Think of alternative forms of exercise, such as tossing a ball, dancing, or rhythm exercises, if a person is hesitant to go out for walks alone (even if he previously thoroughly enjoyed going for long and daily walks). Think about going to a shopping mall where the person can walk safely with you. Bring along two friends. One can walk with your loved one, and the other can sit with you where your loved one can still see you. This gives you a respite and also provides the necessary exercise for the person with Alzheimer's disease.

* Be alert for a loss of control when going up or down stairs. Stumbling can become a dangerous problem.

* Register yourself and the person with Alzheimer's disease in the Alzheimer's Association's Safe Return Program.

7. Senses in the Early-to-Mild Stage

THE SENSES OF TOUCH, vision, and hearing generally remain intact the longest. As people grow older, their ability to hear, see, feel, taste, and smell changes. Usually, one or more of these senses are diminished in people with dementing illnesses.

Keep the senses alive:

* Continue to give your loved one hugs and kisses or intimate touches if this attention had been welcomed before the onset of Alzheimer's disease.

* Stimulate the senses through art, music, gardening, nature, cooking, and other activities.

* Individuals can find comfort in silence and religious practices.

* Touch the arm or hand gently to gain attention, while saying the person's name several times. Be careful not to startle the person.

* Speak directly to the person with Alzheimer's disease. Avoid talking to everyone except the person with Alzheimer's disease. It shows a lack of respect for the dignity of that person. This is not always easy to do, especially if the person with Alzheimer's disease sits quietly. Sadly, one can forget that he is there.

* Enhance visual enjoyment by attending to lighting, and using colors and visual contrasts between floors and walls. Inadequate levels of light can affect a person's ability to concentrate.

* Check all rooms in your home to be sure they are adequately lit. Replace low-wattage light bulbs with brighter ones. This is particularly helpful during the winter months, when the sun may not shine as brightly.

* Check your outside lighting. Light sensors that turn on as someone approaches your home are very useful.

* Be attentive to patterned tile floors that can look like steps and cause a person to trip. Glare from direct sunlight or a highly polished floor can also cause difficulty.

* Play music that will stimulate, excite, or calm the person with Alzheimer's disease.

* Decorate the dinner table three or four times a week and prepare a meal that you know the person will enjoy. This appeal to the senses enhances the quality of life for yourself as well as for the person with dementia.

* Investigate the Alzheimer's Association Memories in the Making Program, which encourages persons with Alzheimer's disease to paint and draw, even if this was not part of their experience in the past. These beautiful drawings can illustrate the dignity within these individuals.

CHAPTER III

Moderate Stage: So Many Changes

Scenario

You and your father have decided to go out to eat at a favorite restaurant, Alexander's Delight. It is his 86th birthday. You walk in the door and ask for a special table reserved near the back of the room and next to the wall. The surroundings will be a little quieter there.

You ask the waiter for your reserved table, and tell the waiter that this is your dad's 86th birthday. Your dad says, "You don't have to tell everybody that it's my birthday. I'm not getting that old. Let's just keep it quiet."

The waiter comes to take your orders. Your dad says, "Give me a hamburger and some spiders." The waiter looks at your dad and says, "Pardon me, Sir. What did you say?" Your dad says, "I want a hamburger and some spiders." You step in and say, "Dad will have the hamburger and french fries." The waiter gives you a knowing nod and continues to fill the order.

Your dad's behavior has been changing. He is more anxious when he is out in public, and he does not want to do as many things as he did before. Still, he knows what he wants, but he no longer remembers words for some things.

Overview of the Moderate Stage

WHO COULD HAVE ANTICIPATED the new challenges and rewards that would come from being a caregiver to a person in the

Moderate stage of Alzheimer's disease? Your strongest awareness may be that life as you had pictured it for you and your loved one is taking a different course. So many abilities seem to have been lost. Yet, so many remain. Focusing on what remains will give the caregiver clues to knowing how to bring happiness and comfort into the life of the person with Alzheimer's disease. Whatever changes you are dealing with, remind yourself that the disease is taking over, and the changes in the person for whom you are caring are not willful acts or done on purpose.

Self-reflection remains throughout the disease, but comes and goes quickly. A nurse said: "Think of Alzheimer's disease like a piece of Swiss cheese. Sometimes there is great clarity and the person can see through the holes; other times things are cloudy and the person cannot understand or reflect."

Changes in the Brain in the Moderate Stage

AS ALZHEIMER'S DISEASE progresses to the Moderate stage, the destruction spreads over the parietal lobes of the brain. When this occurs, the person loses the ability to integrate visual, sound (auditory), and body sensation information.

* In the Moderate stage of Alzheimer's disease, despite the losses, many skills remain, especially judgment, social skills, and the ability to do some complex tasks. Caregivers should focus on maintaining these and other remaining functions.

* At this stage, the individual has trouble dressing, gets lost or is disoriented, and cannot figure out how to use objects.

* The person generally also has great difficulty asking for things (or for help), because the destructive process of Alzheimer's disease has already devastated the temporal lobe speech areas.

* In this stage of the disease, driving can be problematic, because reaction time is often diminished, and the per-

son cannot integrate all the visual and sound information of the environment with the proper body response for the steering wheel and foot pedals.

At this time, patients generally consult physicians for evaluation. When the parietal lobes become involved by the Alzheimer's disease destructive process, the frontal lobe compensatory mechanisms are no longer sufficient, and family members and acquaintances become aware that problems requiring medical evaluation exist.

Tips to Assist the Caregiver in the Moderate Stage

THE CAREGIVER NOW moves into a more extensive phase of involvement with the person who has Alzheimer's disease. The caregiver must realize that more and more activities exist that the person cannot do alone. Extra resources and personnel are needed to continue giving quality care and providing an appropriate level of safety. Instead of being an advocate for the loved one, you become the negotiator.

* You observe that, as much as you would like your loved one to have complete control over her life, more and more situations call for you to become actively involved.

* Behavior problems, such as wandering and agitation, may occur at this time, and the person will need more intensive supervision. When you observe an inappropriate behavior, try to figure out its meaning. Think about what the person is trying to say or do. It is not unusual for agitated behaviors to become worse later in the day or early evening.

* As a caregiver, especially a spouse, you may become cranky, say genuinely mean things, and give help grudgingly. It's important to explain to the person with Alzheimer's disease why you're cranky—probably from a lack of sleep—and why you say mean things. Most likely, you are angry at the disease, not your

spouse. It helps to keep clearing the air and going on as carefully as you both can. In this stage of the disease, you may find that you are caught between balancing your own needs and the needs of the person for whom you are caring.

* Be ready for your own denial, as well as the denial expressed by your loved one or other family members, especially when adjustments and transitions in living arrangements are necessary.

* Learn how to cope with your own anger and hurt feelings, and seek the help of others if you can no longer be objective about a situation. Sometimes the person with dementia will get angry with her spouse or children and blame them for things they haven't done. Insensitive remarks unwittingly can be made.

* Reflect on the way you respond to the person with Alzheimer's disease. If the person becomes combative, ask yourself these questions: "Am I in any danger?" "Can I handle this situation?" Often, you can avoid harm by simply taking five steps back and standing away from the person for a short time. On the other hand, if the person is headed out of the house and onto a busy street, you need to be more aggressive to keep him safe.

* Reach out and rely on outside resources and experts. Delegating tasks to others will help you preserve the strength and energy that will be needed as your loved one progresses into the next stage of the disease.

* Consider having family forums, during which you inform family members of the arrangements that previously have been made regarding emergencies and finances. If no such arrangements have been made, do not delay in doing so now. Make a plan and keep family informed of the arrangements.

* Do not allow daily frustrations and stress to cause you to over-react. Focus on the fact that the disease is caus-

ing the person to behave in this manner, and the person is not doing it purposefully.

* Remove yourself from the caring situation when you find you need respite or have lost your focus or balance.

1. Memory in the Moderate Stage

CONVERSATIONS DURING THIS stage can be difficult, because the person with Alzheimer's disease no longer remembers thoughts long enough to express them or to recall questions long enough to answer them. Although short-term memory may have disappeared in your loved one, long-term memory may be intact. These tips can assist the caregiver.

Stimulate memories:

* Accept wholeheartedly that the person for whom you are caring may not remember from one hour to the next, or from day-to-day, what is on an agenda, what travel plans have been made, where common things such as dishes, pans, and cutlery are located. You may have to repeat plans frequently.

* Create opportunities to reflect on life. Go through old photo albums and talk about happy and enjoyable events.

* Play the beanbag game. Place two chairs about 5 or 6 feet apart, facing each other. The caregiver sits in one chair, and the person with Alzheimer's disease sits in the other. The caregiver tosses the bean bag and, at the same time, asks the person with Alzheimer's disease a simple question that can be answered in one or two words. The beanbag is then tossed back to the caregiver, and the action is repeated. Vary the game by inviting the person with Alzheimer's disease to ask the caregiver a question.

* Sing familiar songs that evoke old memories and feelings.

* Label plants, objects, drawers, to give the person cues to help remember information that came so readily in the past. Being able to name things allows the person more independence. Use large, bold labels that are easy to read.

Embrace memories that remain:

* It can rattle and scare a caregiver when the person for whom they are caring can no longer follow even the simplest of directions. This doesn't necessarily happen gradually. All of a sudden, you're aware that when you say something as simple as, "Put this out in the garbage," he does not understand what you mean and simply can't carry out the direction. In the face of this loss, it's normal to become genuinely exasperated. Only when you gradually realize the ramifications of this loss will you find yourself more creatively dealing with it. Don't stop giving directions. Just remember that, with a short-term memory loss, you may need to help him carry out the task, or to eliminate some of the steps of the task. Keep tasks simple.

* While you should honestly acknowledge to the person with Alzheimer's disease that she has a memory problem, confronting her with her loss of ability only serves to lessen her sense of dignity and self-esteem. Try to remind the person how much she can still do and that she is still loved and valued.

2. Language in the Moderate Stage

COMMUNICATION BETWEEN THE caregiver and the person with dementia is an extremely important—and often difficult—part of the caregiving process. Many times, persons in the Moderate stage of the disease become angry or agitated because they do not understand what is expected of them. They may be frustrated by their inability to make themselves understood. Be aware that some people at this stage may repeat the same sounds or statements or revert to their original language when trying to communicate. Attempt to understand. Be aware also that, at this stage, some people with Alzheimer's disease may insert the wrong word in a sentence. For example, the person may state, "I want to eat my hair," instead of, "I want to comb my hair." Show that you do understand, and do not make a big deal about correcting him. Use these tips to assist the person with dementia as the disease progresses.

Create a positive environment:

* Allow the person to tell stories even if he repeats the same story over and over.

* Avoid expressions that can be taken too literally like "shake a leg" or "jump into bed."

* Never argue with a person with dementia. He will only become angry, more confused, and frustrated. Think about the point you are arguing about and ask yourself, "Is it life threatening?" "Is the argument about going out onto a busy street during rush hour?" If it is, then you must keep safety needs in mind. But if it is over whether the pants he is wearing are black or navy, then don't waste your time or energy.

* Listen sensitively to laments like, "It's so hard!", "I don't know what's going on!", "I don't know what to do!" and commiserate with the confusion the person is feeling. If possible, laugh together about how ridiculous life can be.

* Attempt to be at eye level when you speak with the person with dementia.

* Use short, simple sentences expressing one main idea; avoid complex language, because persons with dementia may have trouble understanding. Pause between sentences and allow plenty of time for the information to be understood.

* Always approach the person slowly and face her when speaking. Be aware of your facial expressions, because she may interpret your mood from your expression, especially if you are frustrated with her behavior.

* Try to eliminate background noise and have conversations in quiet environments to prevent the person with dementia from being distracted and receiving confusing messages.

* Take whatever time is needed to respond to what the person with dementia is trying to articulate, ask, or share verbally. It can become a frustrating guessing game until the information is finally grasped. Despite the difficulty, it is important to maintain communication.

* Use a nondemanding approach—try humor and cheerfulness; humor or a gentle tease often helps caregivers through difficult moments. Convincing someone to get out of bed or to the bathroom is usually easier if you can make a game or joke of it.

* Win a person's trust first. This can often make a task much simpler. One way of doing this is to spend some time chatting before approaching the task at hand. Spend time talking about the weather, or family members, or some reassuring topic, to help get the person in a relaxed frame of mind.

* Remember that, as persons become more impaired, they lose the ability to understand words. Thus, you may need to say, "Here is your soup at this table," instead of "It's time for lunch." They may also revert to words from childhood or earlier in life, so that "Do you need to go to the bathroom?" may not be understood as easily as "Do you have to pee?"

* Talk in a warm, easy-going, pleasant manner. Try to use a tone of voice that you would like people to use with you.

* Keep the pitch of your voice low. Sometimes, when a person doesn't immediately understand, there is a tendency to shout. This will simply upset the person with dementia and will make communication more difficult.

* Redirect the person with dementia if she becomes agitated by moving to another activity or conversation, thereby removing the situation that is causing agitation. Look for the causes of the agitation.

3. Complex Tasks in the Moderate Stage

BECAUSE THE PROGRESSION of the disease is relentless, each day brings change. Caregivers must be constantly on the alert and able to deal with the fact that what worked yesterday may not work today. Reconsidering options and coming up with new approaches, in the face of continuous changes, are part of the hard work that defines caregiving.

Sometimes a caregiver asks a person with dementia to do a task that seems simple to the caregiver but to the person with Alzheimer's disease is overwhelmingly difficult. Getting dressed or brushing teeth are examples of tasks that are very complex because of the many steps involved. Let the person with Alzheimer's disease do as much as possible for himself.

Simplify and be patient:

* Break tasks down into small, concrete steps to enable the person to continue to do the task successfully. Make sure the person is doing one small step at a time. Sometimes caregivers combine several steps together, not realizing the person may no longer be able to do two or three steps at one time.

* Always allow enough time to get dressed or to get ready to go out. It is important not to rush the person with dementia, because that can cause agitation.

* Use simple-to-manage clothing (tube socks that can't be put on the wrong way or slippers with Velcro closings). Purchase clothing items that close in the front or have Velcro fasteners for ease in dressing.

* Try to focus on the familiar tasks that the person did before the onset of the illness, such as washing and drying dishes, making beds, folding laundry, garden-

ing, and the like. People with dementia gradually lose their ability to learn new tasks or skills.

Adjust the environment:

* Keep a spare set of dentures and periodically check for proper fit.

* Use a childproof latch on the refrigerator and cabinet drawers if necessary.

* Consider a ramp with handrails rather than steps.

* Remove knobs from the stove for safety reasons.

* Check containers when disposing of trash, because the person with dementia might have thrown away something valuable.

* Remove fuel sources from patio equipment and grills when not in use.

* Remove scatter rugs and throw rugs to avoid the possibility of slipping or falling.

* Remove wastebaskets in the bathroom and bedrooms, because the person with dementia may mistake them for a toilet.

* Keep laundry and cleaning products in a locked cabinet.

* Keep medications out of reach, and get into a routine of dispensing them at the same time, mornings and evenings.

* Help the person take her medications by having her drink an 8- to 10-ounce glass of cool water each time pills are taken. Initially, she may not want to finish the glass, but keep gently insisting and gradually she will get used to drinking the whole glass.

* Notice if the person is experiencing swallowing difficulties. If so, obtain an evaluation from his physician.

* Consider safety at all times. Does the person need to sit to bathe or dress? Is the person capable of shaving

safely? If so, install appropriate adaptive equipment for the bathroom (bathtub benches, handheld shower heads, grab bars, elevated toilet seats). Consult with an occupational therapist for bathroom adaptations. You can ask your physician for a referral.

4. Social Skills in the Moderate Stage

THE PERSON IN THE Moderate stage of Alzheimer's disease may not understand what is going on in a social setting. The person may want to engage with others, but is uncertain how to accomplish this, so she withdraws or simply sits and stares. A confusing or an overstimulating environment can cause withdrawal. Consider the following tips:

Inform and prepare family and friends:

* Think about the best time for family gatherings. Daytime events are preferable to evening visits. When celebrating special occasions, think about how to include the person with Alzheimer's disease, to keep the sense of family togetherness.

* Alert family members and friends about any memory, behavior, or personality changes in your loved one. You may want to suggest appropriate times to visit, and appropriate activities, such as a ride in the car, or gifts that the loved one would appreciate.

* Encourage family and friends to visit, even if it is challenging for them.

* Keep distractions down to a minimum during the visit. A few people at a time are preferable to a large group.

* Remember that people with dementia have memory loss and may feel humiliated or angry if you ask questions they can no longer answer. Try rephrasing. For example, instead of saying, "Who is this in the picture?" say, "This must be your daughter." This approach allows the person to reply gracefully even if he is not sure and keeps dignity in the interaction.

* Arrange for someone to stay with your loved one if you have to be away. Select someone the person is comfortable with and that you trust to stay with him. Tell your loved one where you're going and how long you'll be gone. You might also take a cell phone along to call, so that he knows that you are coming back.

* Encourage friends and family to call the person with dementia regularly at a scheduled time. Keep conversations short, and tap into events from the past that the person might easily remember. Have a conversation after the phone call to continue to stimulate her memory. You might show her a picture of the caller and talk about the relationship.

* Give appropriate gifts to the person with Alzheimer's disease. Suggestions include favorite foods, pill crushers, books on tape, gift certificates to a hair salon or for a manicure, and home-made certificates good for a car ride or walk.

* Encourage socialization by giving tickets to a concert or musical, sports event, or the circus.

Make adjustments for dining:

* If you are eating lunch at home, and you are having sandwiches, place pieces of fresh fruit on the table also. Invite the person with Alzheimer's disease to join you in eating the fruit with or after the sandwiches.

* Help the person with Alzheimer's disease choose an entrée when dining in a restaurant. This may take patience on the part of the caregiver, because the person initially may not want help. The most successful way is to gently point to different dishes, read the descriptions aloud, and go back and forth with possibilities until she is satisfied with a choice. Even if you're dining with other guests, there is no need to hurry the process. It's amazing how kind others are when they notice that

help is needed. Tell the waiter or waitress your loved one's choice when you're giving yours.

* Fill glasses half-full. It may be necessary to put foam rubber around utensils to give the person with dementia a better grip.

* Serve food in a pie plate or other dish that has a lip on it. This will facilitate getting the food on the spoon or fork more easily, and the food will not slide off the plate.

* Keep finger food available and in sight for easy snacking. Be sure the items are nutritious and in bite-size pieces. The person with Alzheimer's disease may not ask for food when hungry, but the sight of these items will remind the person to eat.

5. Judgment/Reasoning in the Moderate Stage

AS THE CAREGIVER to someone in the Moderate stage of Alzheimer's disease, keep monitoring your frustration level. This is harder than most caregivers can imagine. Anger is an all too common emotion in the caregiver because of the unpredictability of day-to-day circumstances.

Empower your loved one:

* Be alert that your loved one may have faulty judgment regarding safety issues.

* Accept the concerns and worries expressed by persons with dementia. Acknowledge previous discussions and assure them that you will help them with their concerns.

* Help them grieve over any loss of independence. Talk about their concerns and reassure them of your love.

* Cover or take down mirrors if persons are confused by seeing their own image.

* Limit TV viewing if some programs cause confusion. Persons with Alzheimer's disease may think that what is on the screen is happening in reality.

* Seek medical help if persons are having hallucinations.

When I hit the wall, I turned toward the Alzheimer's Chapter
                                        —Sheila Bracken, Caregiver

6. Ambulation in the Moderate Stage

THE PERSON IN the Moderate stage of Alzheimer's disease often can still move around well, however safety issues can be a concern. It will be important to keep the living environment hazard free, well lit, and as accessible as possible. Schedule times for exercise to maintain fitness. Wandering can be a problem, and perceptual-motor problems can affect ambulation.

Adjust to their needs:

* Try closing off part of the house if the physical space is just too confusing for the person with dementia.

* Try removing furniture that is no longer being used. Remove objects if too much clutter is present in the environment.

* Make sure the walking areas are uncluttered and well lit.

* Provide a safe area for the person to walk. If a person tends to wander, clear a pathway through the house. Place chairs at intervals to allow for rest. Remove throw rugs that might cause the person to stumble. Whenever possible, simplify the environment so that the confused person is not too overwhelmed. Consultation with an

occupational therapist for a home safety evaluation can be useful.

* Prompt the person first whenever you plan to move from room to room. Begin with a comment such as, "We need to get up now." Then, gently assist the person to get out of the chair or move across the room; don't just pull or push the person from place to place.

* Provide suggestions and structure. Don't ask if a person wants to do something, instead, say, "It's time to . . . "

* Try to arrange hospitalizations to avoid overnight stays. It is better to take the person home and have in-home assistance than to have him stay in an unfamiliar place. If an overnight stay is necessary, bring familiar items with you like a blanket, pictures, favorite music, or a favorite book. This will help to raise the comfort level and reduce agitation for the person.

* Try to stick with familiar places when traveling. Ask a companion to travel with you to help with the supervision of your loved one. Keep your vacations simple, slow paced, and consider taking several short trips rather than one long trip.

* Be flexible with time schedules. Leave enough slack time for the person to get ready. Allow the person to adjust to any change in schedule. Travel during less busy times of the day.

* Carry information stating that you are traveling with a person with dementia, and list contacts should anything happen to you. Always have identification on your loved one.

* Contact the Alzheimer's Association and enroll your loved one in the Safe Return Program. Have her wear a medical alert identification bracelet. Some chapters have grants to provide these medical alert identifiers free of charge. Consider getting a companion medical alert bracelet for you to wear.

* Bring along items such as familiar pictures, tapes, books, or simple games to distract the person if she becomes agitated when traveling.

* Plan ahead for restroom breaks when traveling or going to appointments. If the person is the opposite sex of the caregiver, you may want to have a companion of the same sex as the person with dementia go along to assist in the restroom.

* Purchase an exercise video produced for the impaired or chair bound person; encourage him to continue exercising.

7. Senses in the Moderate Stage

DESPITE DECREASES IN memory, judgment, and the ability to learn new tasks, persons with dementia still retain senses such as hearing, taste, smell, sight, and the sense of touch. Some senses, such as hearing and sight, may be impaired. Focus on the healthy senses to continue to bring pleasure to persons with dementia.

Stimulate the Senses:

* Touch your loved one often to show that you care, even when your words are no longer understood. Some people shy away from being touched, but most find a gentle touch reassuring.

* Keep your loved one from becoming dehydrated. Many persons with dementia do not get enough fluids, because they no longer recognize the sensation of thirst or they forget to drink. Symptoms of dehydration include dizziness, skin that appears dry, flushing and fever, rapid pulse, confusion, and a refusal to drink.

* Keep a calm environment. Persons with dementia have trouble coping with the stress of a busy environment. When too much is going on in the environment, such as music during conversation or a crowd of people,

persons with dementia can respond with anger or frustration. To understand a response of anger or frustration by your loved one, consider whether it is too noisy or if the group was too large.

* Keep laughter and humor in the relationship. Stories about family and friends and cartoons in daily newspapers are a resource. Read materials aloud to the person for whom you are caring.

* Remember the joy a live animal or bird can bring to someone. Many assisted-living facilities have pet therapy programs or house their own pets or birds to stimulate loving interactions.

* Invite a family minister, priest, rabbi, or spiritual director to contact the person with the disease.

* Be aware that some people in this stage attempt to touch everything in sight and can put items in their mouths inappropriately. This can be a safety issue. Look at the environment as if you were child-proofing a house. Remove anything that could be unsafe or swallowed.

CHAPTER IV

Severe Stage: Making Every Moment Count

Scenario

You and your father have decided to go out to eat at a favorite restaurant, Alexander's Delight. It is his 90th birthday. He has moved from his home to an assisted-living facility, but his Alzheimer's disease has progressed to the point that he will soon need to move to a nursing home that can give him more skilled care.

Your dad still likes to go for rides and sometimes for an ice cream cone. Because it is his 90th birthday, you want to make it very special for him. You decide to take him to Alexander's Delight one more time.

Your dad is in a wheelchair now, so you have asked for a special table that is in a private location in the restaurant. The waiter has come to take your orders.

Your dad has been having some trouble swallowing, so you want him to pick something that will be easy for him to swallow. You ask your dad, "Dad, what do you want to order?"

He says, "You order."

You order the dinner, and you begin to start a conversation with your dad. He becomes agitated watching the people come in and out, and the restaurant is nosier than usual. You can see it is best to cancel your order and leave. You drive through a Dairy Queen and get ice cream for your dad. He is content as you go for a little ride.

Overview of the Severe Stage

THE CAPACITY TO deal with anything complicated is diminished in the Severe stage. Generally, other bodily functions become weak and are failing. Comfort and cleanliness is of great importance.

The overall goal for caregivers and family members is to continue to give loved ones the dignity and respect they deserve. Those who live and work with persons in the Severe stage of the disease must "read" body language as well as listen attentively to any words that are expressed in order to accommodate their loved ones' wishes. This process takes time and patience. Caregivers and family members must slow down and pay attention.

Changes in the Brain in the Severe Stage

IN THE SEVERE STAGE of Alzheimer's disease, the devastation moves into the frontal lobes. Once the frontal lobes are damaged, the person loses the ability to interact properly. At this stage, many persons can no longer be managed by caregivers at home. They lose judgment, reasoning, and social skills, and at this stage respond inappropriately and unacceptably, having lost much of their "civilized" behavior.

In the Severe stage of Alzheimer's disease, many of the brain functions have been consumed. Rather than focus on what is missing, caregivers can focus on helping maintain the remaining functions.

At varying times in the frontal lobe stage, the person can be violent with rages or docile, apathetic, and immobile. Touching, such as helping the person undress, can trigger violence to repel the contact, possibly injuring either the caregiver or the person with Alzheimer's disease. In the end stages, the destructive Alzheimer's disease process has killed nearly all the nerve cells of the cerebral hemispheres except the strip of motor cortex and the visual cortex, which is why in nursing homes, the main activity seems to be walking and pacing. In the final stages, even these brain areas are destroyed, and the individual will be bedridden and relatively unresponsive.

Tips to Assist the Caregiver in the Severe Stage

THE CAREGIVER IS NOW moving into the third phase of involvement with the person who has Alzheimer's disease. You will find yourself using a direct, authoritative approach.

* You need to take the lead in making most of the decisions regarding the welfare of the person for whom you are caring. You will need to keep your own health and energy level high, so that you can respond to the rapidly changing needs of the person with Alzheimer's disease.

* The extreme difficulty in communicating is frustrating for both the caregiver and the person with Alzheimer's disease. It is critically important that, as a caregiver, you continue to talk to your loved one about the food, the weather, the place, someone you've been with, upcoming events like doctor appointments, a social activity, or current news. Focus on ways to keep the person in touch with what is going on.

* In this final phase, you may be dealing with finances and alternative housing, as well as insurance issues. Hopefully, you will have previously discussed end-of-life issues with the person who has Alzheimer's disease. You may find it difficult to accept the fact that your loved one no longer recognizes you.

The caregiver can consider these tips when working with the person in the Severe Stage of Alzheimer's disease:

* Talk in a slow, controlled manner to the person with dementia even if he does not respond. Your voice can be a comfort.

* Concentrate on caring for the person with dignity. Be attentive to dress and surroundings, even as the body loses control of functions.

* Take time to listen.

* Remember that the person for whom you are caring is in control of accepting or rejecting the food, help, comfort you want to give. Caregivers are in control of cleanliness, the person's safety needs, and listening and watching to discern the loved one's wishes.

* Acquaint hospital staff with the person's abilities and habits. Try to arrange any hospitalizations to avoid overnight stays. It would be better to take the person home and have in-home assistance than to stay in an unfamiliar place. If a stay is necessary, bring familiar items with you, such as a blanket, pictures, favorite music, or a favorite book. This helps put everyone more at ease and reduces the possibility of agitation.

* Consider the option of hospice care. Hospice care can be delivered in the home, at a nursing facility, or at a residence such as a hospice house.

* Take time to be with the person who is receiving hospice care. Hold the person's hand, kiss her on the cheek, rub or pat her hand . . . anything to let the person know that you are present.

The word "hospice" comes from the Latin word hospes *meaning "guest." It was used in the Middle Ages to refer to a lodging place where sick and weary travelers stopped to refresh themselves. The word was applied to care for dying patients in 1967, when Dr. Cicely Saunders established St. Christopher's Hospice, in a suburb of London. The first hospice in the United States was established in New Haven, Connecticut, in 1974. Hospice has come to mean both a place and a philosophy for the care of the terminally ill and their families. The care aims at relieving pain and other distress—not curing the illness.*

1. Memory in the Severe Stage

IN THE SEVERE STAGE of Alzheimer's disease, even long-term memory fails. It is still possible, however, to trigger some memory with pictures and sounds, bringing enjoyment to both the caregiver and the person with Alzheimer's disease.

Go with the flow:

* Be prepared to deal with the fact that the person with Alzheimer's disease may fluctuate in and out of lucid moments. He may not recognize you, or may call you by another's name. He will vary in responsiveness. If you are prepared for this, you will be better able to go-with-the-flow.

2. Language in the Severe Stage

COMMUNICATION WILL BE very difficult at this stage, and therefore it will be hard to determine how much comprehension remains. Never assume the person does not understand your words of comfort and assurance even if she does not respond. The person may recognize statements or movements. Caregivers should look for new ways to communicate using all the senses.

Read nonverbal cues:

* Accept and expect communication to consist of single words or gestures.

* Be attuned to nonverbal communication such as closing the lips tightly to refuse food or pulling on clothing indicating anxiety or pain.

* Be alert to any type of communication.

3. Complex Tasks in the Severe Stage

IN THE LAST STAGE of Alzheimer's disease, plaques and tangles (hardened areas of brain tissue that are the physical traces of the disease process) are widespread throughout the brain. In the Severe stage of Alzheimer's disease, a person may be bed-ridden much or all of the time. The ability to do complex tasks has faded, and the person is mostly dependent on others for care.

Alleviate fears and stress:

* Remove or hide locks with tape, especially in the bath-room, so that the person with dementia does not lock himself in. Alternatively, remove the doors and use curtains for privacy.

* Be conscious of the person's needs during bath time. Bath time can be very difficult, because the person with dementia may have become fearful of water. If possible, the caregiver can get into the shower with the person. Also, to alleviate fear of water, a bath or shower chair in a tub can be used. Flexible hand-held shower nozzles can be used to bathe the person. This will eliminate getting down into the tub which, in some cases, can cause extreme agitation. Also, use a shower chair in the shower.

* Plan to unwrap gifts for the person with dementia and then explain and show the purpose of the gift.

* Encourage as much independence as possible with any abilities that remain.

4. Social Skills in the Severe Stage

IN THE SEVERE STAGE, persons tend to withdraw from social interaction and may have lost a sense of self. Other symptoms include increased sleep time and incontinence.

Let go of expectations:

* Provide extra time for eating, because it will take the person with dementia longer to consume a meal.

* Approach holidays as a new adventure. Start new traditions that incorporate the individual's remaining skills in activities during family gatherings. This is especially helpful if the person with Alzheimer's disease can no longer participate in traditional activities during family gatherings.

* Ask a friend to help, if decorating or purchasing gifts is too difficult for you.

* Tell your family and friends that it is important for you to talk about your loved one, because they may be reluctant to mention her for fear of upsetting you. Share stories with the rest of the family and be creative with your grief.

* Set realistic expectations. Recognize that holidays may be a difficult time and plan accordingly. Set limits about what you can and cannot do. Ask yourself, "Am I doing what I want to do or what I think others want me to do?" Remember, at this stage in the caregiving process, it is important to take care of yourself. Save your energy to keep your balance, so that you can enjoy other people in your life who love you.

5. Judgment/Reasoning in the Severe Stage

IN THE SEVERE STAGE, the individual with dementia lacks the abilities necessary to have sound judgment or reasoning.

Carry out their wishes:

* Keep documents concerning the person's end-of-life wishes readily available.

* Carry emergency contact information in your car, on your person either in a pocket or a purse, and displayed

in an obvious site within your home in case of emergency.

* Keep a cell phone with you at all times in case of an emergency.

Make adjustments for changes in sexual behavior:

* Try to anticipate bodily needs. If the person starts to undress, or pulls at clothes, consider that the person cannot verbalize the need to use the toilet, go to bed, or is too hot or in pain.

* Do not overreact, become angry, or make fun of the behavior if the person is engaging in unusual behavior with the genitals. Try to assess the situation. Perhaps the person needs to use the toilet, or clothes may be too tight. Maybe the person wants to go to bed but cannot verbalize this. Gently redirect the person's activity. If sexual issues continue to be a problem, seek outside help.

* Gently redirect the person when actions such as fondling, or grabbing a woman's breast, or attempting sexual intimacy occur. If gentle redirection is not possible, seek outside help.

* Try to distract the person with another activity, perhaps in an adjoining room, if the person becomes agitated when you try to get her to discontinue the behavior.

* Purchase appropriate materials, such as mattress protectors, flannel-coated rubber pads, and other materials available at your pharmacy when incontinence occurs.

* Review the web sites recommended in Section C for additional information regarding sexuality and intimacy issues.

6. Ambulation in the Severe Stage

AT THIS STAGE, wandering and agitation are a common problem. The person can have significant difficulty getting in or out of chairs, and may become bedridden. A lack of mobility may lead to skin breakdown and pressure sores. This is the time to focus on what the person is still able to do or enjoy.

Be creative:

* Place the bed mattress and springs on the floor to protect the person with dementia from injury, if falling out of bed could be a problem. This can also decrease roaming.

* Place the person who is bedridden near a window in order to enjoy looking outdoors.

* Find ways to fulfill the person's desire to be out of doors, even if you have to push her bed out on a patio.

* Have available familiar lap robes, warm socks, and blankets to provide comfort if circulation is poor.

* Learn about proper positioning of the immobile person to prevent skin breakdown.

* Consult hospice workers for additional ways to provide movement for the person for whom you are caring.

7. Senses in the Severe Stage

ALTHOUGH THE LOSS of reasoning, judgment, and social skills occurs, the senses remain fairly intact. A caregiver is challenged at this time to "read" body language. Your voice, or touch, can be reassuring and will let the person know of your presence.

Communicate through the senses:

* Touch the person in any way acceptable to him, such as combing his hair or gently stroking his arm or chest.

* Use hand and body lotion and massage the person's hands and feet and arms. Be sensitive to any fragrances that might no longer be pleasing to the person and avoid such scented products.

* Encourage frequent visits by anyone who will connect with the person and relieve loneliness.

* Comfort individuals in this stage of dementia by giving them cuddly stuffed animals and soft pillows and afghans to stimulate the sense of touch.

* Comfort the person with music or pleasant sounds. Although the person may not be able to speak, he may be comforted by hearing sounds.

* Provide liquids, malts, or anything compatible with the person's diet and swallowing capabilities for her to enjoy. Enjoyment of the taste of sugar may still be present.

* Give liquids by means of an oral syringe when the person with Alzheimer's disease can no longer suck on a straw or swallow.

* Make the living atmosphere aesthetically pleasing by using pleasant colors, pictures, and sounds.

* Accommodate the person's spiritual needs.

Ethicist Gilbert Meilaender wrote recently in a paper presented to his colleagues on the President's Council on Bioethics, "One might take the living body, not the immaterial will or the power of choice, as the locus of personal presence." We are not minds alone or bodies alone, but embodied souls and ensouled bodies. To understand this truth is to understand the dignity of those whose minds are fading, but whose presence as persons can never be in doubt.
—"The Human Face of Alzheimer's"
by Colleen Carroll Campbell, *The New Atlantis.*

Helpful Information Concerning Alzheimer's Disease or Related Dementia

Questions
and Answers

THIS SECTION CONTAINS information that is not necessarily "stage-specific" according to the disease progression. Many topics could be addressed here, but we have chosen those that seem most important.

Adjusting to Limitations

EVERY DISEASE AFFECTS THE body in some way and leaves the body with limitations. For persons with any disease, the frustration is that no one expects to have to live with limitations. We generally feel that other people can have limitations, but not us—so, learning to live with limitations takes some time for persons with the disease, as well as for caregivers, family members, and friends.

The adjustment time differs for everyone. Sometimes, persons with a disease or limitation adjust more quickly than the rest of the family. Or just the opposite can take place: family members, caregivers, and friends adjust to the idea of changing directions or rethinking dreams before the person with a disease.

Tension occurs during the time of transition, and everyone connected with the family will be expected to make changes. This is a challenging time, because it can bring out the best and the worst in all of us. Here's where impatience and patience are displayed daily. Here's where depression and acceptance weave in and out of the situation.

All humans need to learn to live with limitations through-out their lives, because no one is perfect. But when individuals and their families receive the diagnosis of Alzheimer's disease, fear and dread enter the picture. Pursuing correct information about the disease and how it might affect you or a loved one is most important in alleviating this fear and dread. Each person's life will be affected differently. Some people find skills and abilities they never used or knew they had.

Life can be filled with new ways of living that haven't been tried before. New people will come into your life because of the disease—health professionals, others who have the disease, online buddies found through local Alzheimer's Associations, and others. Unique bonds will be made with others. Blessings may be right around the corner—if we look for them.

Frequently Asked Questions

WE HAVE PUT THE INFORMATION in this section of the book in a "Question and Answer" format so that readers can locate information quickly. As you read this section, keep in mind that the motivating factor is to help persons with Alzheimer's disease have their wishes carried out, to live a happy and full life. In the process, caregivers, family members, and friends will grow in new experiences, and must maintain balance in their lives as they, too, find new ways to live fulfilled, happy lives.

1. When Do You Tell Others?

WHEN DO YOU tell others you or your loved one has Alzheimer's disease?

Tell others that you or your loved one has Alzheimer's disease after a diagnosis has been made by a medical professional—and when you are comfortable doing so.

Unfortunately, in our society a stigma is attached to Alzheimer's disease, just as it is with cancer, AIDS, and many other diseases. Some people do not want to acknowledge that they have the disease, and their families agree that no one will talk about it.

This can cause the person with Alzheimer's disease and his family to feel ashamed. No one is at fault for getting Alzheimer's disease, and no person with Alzheimer's disease or his family should feel ashamed. Medical science does not yet understand how or why people develop Alzheimer's disease. Currently no cure exists for the disease. A definitive diagnosis is still only possible after death.

Admitting to the diagnosis allows a person with Alzheimer's disease and her family to participate in planning for the future. Everyone wants to have as much control over their lives as possible. By telling others about the disease, one can find help from local Alzheimer's Association chapters, state Offices on Aging, and many others who have experience with the disease.

Alzheimer's disease can be diagnosed at many ages. Early-onset Alzheimer's disease affects persons between the age of 30 and 60 years, whereas late-onset Alzheimer's disease is diagnosed in persons 60 years and older.

Acknowledging the disease and planning for the future gives comfort to everyone involved and assures persons with the disease that their desires for their lives will be respected.

2. Long-Distance Care

WHAT SHOULD I DO if the person I'm caring for lives in another state?

At a recent workshop, twenty-six people gathered over their lunch hour to share information and to gain insights into how they can best care for the person who was just diagnosed with Alzheimer's disease. More than half of the people present had a similar concern: "How can I help my loved one who lives in another state?" The concern and love for the person far away was so painful that several people cried as they explained their situation of being too far away to see their loved one on a regular basis.

Problems can go unnoticed unless a close eye is kept on the well-being of the person with Alzheimer's disease. Keeping in touch with the person's physician can be helpful in knowing if any of these physical or mental changes are a cause for concern. If you are many miles away, you can regularly check in with the person's physician. With the physician's help, you can still be present for any major transitional changes that will occur in your loved one's life.

Most of the people present at the workshop were not aware that the Alzheimer's Association has local chapters throughout the United States. Many of the web sites listed in Section C of this book can be helpful, and you will be able to find agencies located in the same state as your loved one. Contact with these agencies can support your efforts in the caregiving process. In addition to the physician, you will then have another contact to help you.

Even at a distance, you can help your loved one with legal and financial matters. Upcoming sections address how to handle these issues. However, as the disease progresses, it may be necessary for the primary caregiver to be nearby.

3. Family Forums

HOW CAN "FAMILY FORUMS" be useful during the caregiving process?

One of the most difficult tasks for families is coming to an agreement on what is the best care for loved ones with Alzheimer's disease. The first task is to discover the wishes of the loved one for his care during the disease process. Early in the process of the disease, the loved one should be encouraged to indicate what his wishes are concerning many things— among them how he would like to be cared for during the progression of the disease. It is important to complete this decision-making in the early stages of the disease, to make certain that family members and friends know the loved one's wishes. This provides the loved one with as much control over his life as possible. The Family Forum is the best way to make sure your loved one's wishes are known.

Some families formalize these forums by inviting key members of the family to a meeting where an agenda covering all topics to be discussed has been prepared. Other forums occur more spontaneously, as people normally gather together for holidays or visits.

The first meeting should look at the facts of what happens during the disease progression and see how the wishes of the loved one can be carried out. It is important to remember, however, that while family members want to be able to honor all the wishes of the loved one, promises should never be made that might not be kept.

During family meetings, it is important that someone be given the authority to carry out the plans for caregiving. Other members will certainly assist in the caregiving responsibilities and can take on the task of financial planning and deal with other issues. The person who is given the responsibility for caregiving should establish a line of communication with other family members to keep them informed of the loved one's progress.

If the person with Alzheimer's disease has children, the responsibilities can be shared. The important thing is that the loved one knows how he is to be cared for.

If only one family member exists, a child or a spouse, then all caregiving responsibilities fall on that individual. However, she can call a Family Forum with other relatives and friends, so that broader groups are involved in the caregiving plans.

When the person with Alzheimer's disease is single, a particularly close relative or friend should take the lead and call a Family Forum for those close to the person. The same process is followed; that is, give the person an opportunity to indicate what he wants concerning care during the disease progression and then determine who has the authority to act in his best interest.

At each stage of the disease, it is important to look at the skills and abilities present in the person with Alzheimer's disease. A number of family meetings will probably occur throughout the disease process. During each stage of the disease (Early-to-Mild stage, Moderate stage, and Severe stage), family members can look at the remaining skills and abilities and discuss creative ways to enhance the quality of life of the person with the disease as well as the primary caregiver.

Family Forums give a person with Alzheimer's disease comfort in knowing she will be cared for by those who have her best interests in mind, and that she will be given the dignity and respect she deserves.

4. Key Financial Issues

WHAT ARE SOME KEY financial issues to consider during the progression of Alzheimer's disease?

About one-fourth of American families are providing care for an older adult, an adult child, or a friend. More than half of caregivers are women, whereas care receivers are about evenly divided between men and women. The typical caregiver is a married woman in her mid-forties who works full-time, is a high school graduate, and has an annual household income of $35,000.

It has been estimated that between 20% and 40% of caregivers are in the "sandwich generation," having children under the age of 18 years to care for in addition to an older relative. The current long-term care system would collapse without family caregivers. In 2004, it was estimated that the contribution of America's caregivers was valued at $257 billion per year.

In a recent Gallup poll, 1 in 10 Americans indicated they had a family member with Alzheimer's disease, and 1 in 3 knew someone with the disease.

The average lifetime cost of caring for a person with Alzheimer's disease is $174,000.

The annual total U.S. cost of caring for individuals with Alzheimer's disease is $100 billion, as estimated by the Alzheimer's Association and the National Institute on Aging.

As many as 7 out of 10 people with Alzheimer's disease are cared for in the home by family and friends, who provide 75% of the direct care. Paying for the other 25% of care costs an average of $12,500 a year, most often coming out of family members' pockets.

The average cost for nursing home care for a person with Alzheimer's disease is $42,000 per year.

Many more statistics are available concerning the cost of care for families with a person diagnosed with Alzheimer's disease. But this brief review shows that caregivers will need to find assistance concerning financial matters throughout the disease progression.

Many persons with the disease believe they have saved for their future and will have the financial resources necessary for care throughout their lifetime. Experience shows that the savings of a person with Alzheimer's disease can become depleted quickly. When that happens, reliance on family finances, and state and federal assistance is necessary for the person who has Alzheimer's disease.

As soon as a family member is diagnosed with the disease, caregivers should facilitate a conversation to plan for the future care of the loved one. The family conversation can take many different turns on this issue, because the care of the total person should be discussed.

This is a suggested list of some financial documents that will help you to take the necessary steps to manage your loved one's financial resources. Review these documents, even if you feel you are already familiar with them, and begin making necessary plans.

* Bank and brokerage account information

* Insurance policies

* Monthly living costs and outstanding bills

* Stock and bond certificates

* Social Security payment information

* Retirement benefits

* Outside income

* Personal property

* Mortgage papers or other ownership papers

A financial planner can help you prepare to fulfill the wishes of the person with Alzheimer's disease, as well as protect the financial position of your own family.

5. Key Legal Issues

WHAT ARE SOME KEY legal issues to consider during the progression of Alzheimer's disease?

The planning process includes attending to legal as well as financial issues. Many communities have lawyers who specialize in elder law, which includes guardianship determination, spousal impoverishment, disability planning, living wills or trusts, and durable powers of attorney.

An attorney also can help determine the competency required to participate in the creation and execution of the documents. The caregiver must help the person with Alzheimer's disease address the following issues:

* Create a durable power of attorney. This document gives authority for decision making in financial matters and/or health care. It has the words " . . . this power of attorney shall not be affected by the subsequent disability or incapacity of the principal," or, " . . . this power of attorney shall become effective upon the disability or incapacity of the principal." If it is not a "durable" power of attorney, it is not effective when the person with Alzheimer's disease becomes legally incapacitated.

* Make a living will. This document describes the end-of-life wishes of the person making the Living Will. It can describe such things as the withholding of life-sustaining treatment. The form of a Living Will varies from state to state in the United States.

* Prepare a will. This document describes what is to be done with a person's property and possessions after death.

To help make this process easier, seek professional advice in these matters. Community agencies, such as the local Chapter of the Alzheimer's Association and other community agencies, have informational materials to guide you. To summarize the legal tasks for caregivers:

* Listen to the person with dementia and assist in carrying out the person's wishes.

* Be open to discussing the future.

* Include other family members in this process, and initiate a Family Forum to let other family members know the wishes of the person with dementia.

* Determine who has the responsibility to care for the person with dementia; always arrange for an alternate.

* Consult a medical professional to help determine legal capacity.

* Determine whether legal documents were executed prior to the diagnosis of Alzheimer's disease.

* Give copies of the Durable Power of Attorney to all designated individuals.

* Provide your physician and other health care providers with a copy of the Durable Power of Attorney and Living Will.

* Create a list of close family members, lawyers, financial planners, and accountants for future reference.

* Inform others where all legal and financial documents are kept, and make sure they are accessible in case of an emergency.

Taking care of financial and legal issues can bring comfort to the person with dementia, family members, and other concerned individuals. Having plans in place to meet the financial and legal needs of the person with Alzheimer's disease allows everyone to focus on the daily issues of care and to find creative ways to add to the dignity of life.

6. Medications and Other Illnesses

WHAT ROLE CAN medications and other illnesses play in the progression of Alzheimer's disease?

People with dementia are very vulnerable to overmedication, to reactions from combinations of drugs, and to the many side effects of various medications (such as falling, drowsiness, tremor, a sudden increase in agitation, and strange move-ments). Confusion and sudden changes in a person's level of functioning can be caused by medication. Tranquilizers and sedatives given to calm behavior or facilitate sleep can affect bladder functioning and cause incontinence.

Many research studies throughout the world involve the use of new and experimental medications for Alzheimer's dis-ease. The caregivers and the person with Alzheimer's disease must evaluate the potential side effects and other pros and cons of participating in such drug trials. Consult the web sites listed in Section C for additional information.

* Acute illness, such as urinary tract infection, pneumo-nia, gastrointestinal infection, or any illness causing a fever, can lead to or increase confusion. Very often, it is difficult to recognize acute illnesses in people with dementia, because they cannot readily verbalize symp-toms. Any sudden changes in behavior may be a signal of an acute illness and should be discussed with a physician.

* Chronic illness such as angina, congestive heart failure, or diabetes can affect a person's mood and level of functioning. Also, chronic pain associated with arthri-tis, ulcers, or headaches can cause irritability.

* Constipation can be very uncomfortable and may con-tribute to behavior changes. To keep bowel movements regular, assist the person with Alzheimer's disease in taking Metamucil, or other stool softeners, with a large glass of water once or twice a day.

* Symptoms of depression, such as impaired concentra-tion, memory loss, apathy, and sleep disturbances, can mimic dementia. It is important for the physician to consider the diagnosis of depression when evaluating a person for Alzheimer's disease or other dementia.

7. Changing Living Circumstances

HOW DO YOU KNOW when it is time to change the living situation for the person with Alzheimer's disease?

Some things to consider in making a decision to change the living situation for the person with Alzheimer's disease are:

* The mental and physical condition and the stage of the disease.

* The overall ability of the primary caregiver to continue to provide care.

* The finances of the loved one and the finances of the caregiver.

Once the diagnosis of Alzheimer's disease or related dementia has been made, a number of resources are available to caregivers: local chapters of the Alzheimer's Association throughout the United States, local Offices on Aging, and health care professionals. Gather information concerning the disease as well as the costs of care.

A family physician once said: "The best way I can help persons who are diagnosed with Alzheimer's disease or related dementia is to help the caregiver throughout the disease process."

Caregivers are key to the decision of changing living situations. Here is an example of how one caregiver, Pat Callone, handled the situation when her father had Alzheimer's disease.

My father lived at home alone until he was 95. Through the Early-to-Mild stage, I was able to get local resources to come to Dad's home. I used the Office on Aging, the local Alzheimer's Association chapter, and the Presbyterian Outreach. The Visiting Nurses Association equipped Dad with an electronic emergency call system for him to wear throughout the home. I called my father twice a day to monitor his activities.

After a stay in the hospital because of a urinary tract infection, physical therapy professionals said Dad should not be home alone because he could not remember to put his hands on the arms of the chair in order to lower his body into it. He couldn't remember the process and would just fall backwards to sit down.

That first move from home to an assisted-living facility that knew how to care for persons with dementia was painful for Dad, my husband, and me. My father did not understand why he needed to leave his beloved home. Attempts to find someone to live with him in his one-level home failed and were too expensive. My husband and I could not take my father into our home because it was a tri-level design and because I needed to work full time. Because of his own physical condition, my husband could not take care of my Dad. The assisted-living facility became "home" to my father after about 6 months.

But he began to have more serious urinary tract infections and developed trouble swallowing. After another stay in the hospital, it was decided that he needed a special diet so that he could continue to eat. The assisted-living facility could not keep Dad, because "assisted living" means that the person can function without a special diet or the need of assistance in self-care. While staying at the assisted-living facility, Dad's finances began to dwindle due to the increased cost of medications and increased cost of care.

The next move was from the assisted-living facility to a well-respected rehabilitation center and nursing home. I contacted the state office that handles Medicaid, explained the situation, and completed the necessary papers so that Dad could receive Medicaid. The stipulation under Medicaid was that my father needed to share a room with another person.

The move from the assisted-living facility where my father was used to having his privacy to the shared bedroom was another difficult move. My husband and I offered to pay for my father's full care from our own financial resources, but a counselor suggested that my dad deserved Medicaid, that the home would give him good care, and that my husband and I needed to save our resources for our own care.

But the living situation did not turn out to be what we had hoped. Dad's greatest pleasure during the day was having a window to look out. Dad loved the window that was next to his bed because he could watch the parking lot and the people go by. I still wanted to move him to a private room, but I also wanted him to have his greatest pleasure—to be able to look out the window and watch the people and cars go by. There were no single rooms available for him with the window view that he had in the shared bedroom.

More infections entered my father's system, and one day the home called me to have Dad taken to the hospital. At the hospital, physicians found that my father had five different infections. One of them was severe enough that his frail body could not combat it.

After a week in the hospital trying to clear the five infections, the family physician met with my husband and me and told us that there was nothing more the health profession could do and that the infections would persist until Dad's death.

Through dialogue with the doctor it was decided that Dad would move to Hospice House. At Hospice House, we were welcomed warmly; arrangements were made by the hospital social worker to have the ambulance take my father from the hospital to Hospice House.

With a Durable Power of Attorney, I completed the necessary paper work that would pay for Dad's care. Hospice took care of making all the arrangements with Medicaid, etc. Nurses, social workers, chaplains and volunteers at Hospice were wonderful to work with.

My father stayed at Hospice House for about 2 months. He began to get better because of the loving care given to him. No more strong antibiotics were put into his system to try to bring him back to health. Hospice care was for comfort until death.

Gradually, my Dad moved into the last part of the Severe stage. He had volunteers to feed him when I could not be there. The Hospice House team also took care of my husband and me. I knew my father was being treated with the respect and dignity he deserved. I was with him at his death, which was quiet and peaceful.

Every family has different concerns and financial resources. Every family needs the assistance of knowledgeable and caring health professionals for guidance. Each time a move occurs, it is usually triggered by a combination of three things:

* The mental and physical condition of the person with Alzheimer's disease.

* The ability of the primary caregiver to continue to provide care into the next stage of the disease.

 * The financial position of the person with Alzheimer's
   disease and caregivers.

The time of disease progression can be long or short, as
determined by the overall health of the person with Alzheimer's disease. Help is available. The most important thing is
to get into a network of health care professionals who are real
"friends" during the progression of the disease. Pat's family
physician, the local chapter of the Alzheimer's Association,
the Visiting Nurses Association, the state Office on Aging,
Hospice House, and volunteer organizations were lifelines for
Pat and her husband.

8. Living Environment

HOW DOES THE living environment affect the person with Alzheimer's disease?

There is a saying: "If you've met one Alzheimer's resident—you've met one Alzheimer's resident." While not particularly humorous, the saying puts into perspective what should
be intuitive when considering all aspects of the life of the
person with Alzheimer's disease, including the living environment. Whether it is an individual's home or a communal living
arrangement, it is actually an environment for an "individual."

Key basic tenets are necessary to make the environment
appropriate for the person with Alzheimer's disease: independence, choice, security, privacy, companionship, stimulation,
and rhythm. Creatively modifying the environment for the
individual, and varying it as the disease progresses, is vital to
utilizing the environment to maximize the potential of persons
with Alzheimer's disease.

 * INDEPENDENCE. Elderly individuals often drive their
   automobiles far longer than safety would allow, as a
   gesture of independence. Becoming dependent on others is a tremendous psychological blow that often results in the deterioration of physical health. The onset
   of dementia generally does not affect our innate need
   for independence. An environment that enables inde-

pendence facilitates an individual's ability to complete activities of daily living and improves physical health.

* CHOICE. Providing choices is critical to maintaining independence. These choices can range from the most mundane to the most complex. Choosing clothes to be worn and properly dressing oneself can mean the difference between a good day and a bad day for the individual. Food choices make a person's meals more palatable and decrease the need for dietary supplements. Allowing the choice of bedroom wall color or window coverings individualizes a person's private space and can help the person more readily identify that space.

* SECURITY. Both mental and physical security are important to individuals and caregivers. Appropriate environmental design can allow independence and still provide safety and security. A comfortable, welcoming environment can diminish agitation, wandering, or rummaging through other individual's belongings.

* PRIVACY. In any living situation that involves others, privacy can be very difficult to provide; however, designing clearly defined spaces that belong to an individual is critical to that person's emotional security. Personal memorabilia should be prominently displayed. Periodically changing the memorabilia can help engage the interest of the individual.

* STIMULATION. Stimulation throughout the environment, from the artwork on the walls, to the style of furniture, to the texture of fabrics, all combine to heighten a person's sense of emotional security and familiarity with the environment. Providing variety in the environment is important to maintain a person's interest in his surroundings. The distinctiveness of a person's private space will reduce the likelihood that others will wander into that space. Exterior spaces provide stimulation and can trigger memories of the sun's warmth, the feel of a breeze on one's face, or the smell of flowers.

* RHYTHM. Each person has her own daily and seasonal rhythm, which includes sleeping, toileting, and eating. Each person's rhythm should be acknowledged, encouraged, and balanced against the rhythm of the caregiver, but never simply modified for the convenience of the caregiver. An environmental design that accommodates individual rhythms without disrupting the rhythms of others can be accomplished by discarding barriers to bathing, toileting, and food preparation without ignoring safety issues.

A successful environment is the result of attention to the smallest detail. The environment must respect individual independence while maintaining security, provide privacy while allowing desired companionship, and provide stimulation while also maintaining an individual's life rhythms.

We should strive never to modify the individual to suit the environment, but instead creatively modify the environment to meet the needs of the individual, so that the environment can enhance the quality of life for the person with Alzheimer's disease.

9. Changing Caregiver Roles

HOW CAN CAREGIVERS to person's with Alzheimer's disease learn to be comfortable in their ever-changing roles?

An effective caregiver is constantly challenged to keep the lines of communication open with the person who has Alzheimer's disease, as well as with concerned family and friends. Some of the skills required of the caregiver include the ability to be attentive to the verbal and nonverbal communication of the loved one, initiate solutions to problems never encountered before, and distinguish facts from feelings.

Because Alzheimer's disease involuntarily changes a person's behavior, the caregiver can easily be overwhelmed and have difficulty understanding the loved one's behavior in a rational way.

Making good decisions requires self-discipline by the caregiver. Self-discipline requires the caregiver to wait and, while waiting, to think about how to act. Usually, these components of self-discipline occur simultaneously. By reflecting on these components, however, three styles used by most decision-makers become apparent. These styles take into consideration the amount of power or control the decision-maker will keep or give away.

When using the first style, the caregiver gives all the power over to the person for whom she is caring. In the second style, the caregiver collaborates with others and makes shared decisions regarding the person for whom she is caring. Finally, in the third style, the caregiver keeps all the power and simply makes the decisions.

The effective caregiver will change the amount of power she retains or gives up as the disease progresses. The healthy caregiver stops and thinks about what is best for herself and for the person for whom she is caring—before responding or acting. Several questions can help the caregiver decide which style to use; the next sections describe the three styles of caring.

Style One

THE CAREGIVER WILL give all the power over to the person being cared for and will act as a resource person for that person. Use this style if you can answer, "Yes" to most of these questions:

* Is the person capable of living independently?
* Do you believe the person will be safe and not be in any harm due to forgetfulness or inability to stay focused?
* Does the person want to help and can he follow directions?
* Is the person able to make sound judgments?
* Is the person generally "aware" even during times of forgetfulness?
* Is the person strong-willed and unable to take direction from others?
* Has the person told you that he is not yet ready for someone to take care of his needs?

❋ Are you able to let go of your opinions and ideas and follow the lead from the person for whom you are caring?

In the Early-to-Mild stage of the disease, most people with Alzheimer's disease will want independence and a caregiver who will act as an advocate and resource. As a caregiver, you can refrain from doing things for a person that she can do for herself, and you can encourage her to be independent as much as possible.

Style Two

THE CAREGIVER WILL collaborate with others and make shared decisions. Use this style if you can answer "Yes" to most of these questions:

❋ Has a diagnosis of Alzheimer's disease been made by a physician with expertise in dementia?

❋ Are you becoming less able to meet the basic needs of the person for whom you are caring?

❋ Do you find yourself becoming overwhelmed or depressed or worried a majority of the time?

❋ Are family members and friends showing concern and asking to be part of the long-term caregiving process?

❋ Are you concerned about the safety needs of the person for whom you are caring?

❋ Has the person with dementia indicated that she would like to go places or do things, but cannot do so independently?

❋ Is there conflict among family members regarding the method of care the person with dementia should receive?

Although a caregiver may be able to answer "Yes" to these questions early on in the progression of the disease, usually in the Moderate stage the need to share the decision-making power becomes apparent. Although you would like your loved one to have complete control over her life, you note that more and more situations call for you to become actively involved. The task of balancing caregiving and your own needs will come into greater conflict. Delegating some of the caregiving to other professionals, friends, and family members will become a necessity. At this stage, you can no longer allow your loved one to have full power over her life, but you don't assume full control either.

Style Three

THE CAREGIVER WILL keep all the power and simply make the decisions. Use this style if you can answer "Yes" to most of these questions:

* Have you been given Durable Power of Attorney—the authority to make decisions for financial matters or health care?

* Are the financial and material resources of the person with Alzheimer's disease becoming depleted?

* Is the person unable to comprehend the contents and implications of signing legal documents?

* Are you, as caregiver, comfortable taking the lead and making difficult decisions?

* Is your judgment clear, and have you taken into consideration the pros and cons of your actions?

* Can you be counted on to act rationally in times of stress or crises?

* Have you informed family members, friends, and other concerned individuals that you are carrying out the wishes of the person with Alzheimer's disease?

This third style can be used when the person with Alzheimer's disease is in the Severe stage. You may also use this style in other stages of the disease process whenever the caregiver is carrying out wishes the loved one has previously discussed.

There is comfort in knowing that, throughout the progression of the disease, only three interactive styles are possible for a caregiver to take. Understanding and using these three styles properly—giving over all control, sharing control, and taking the lead—can be invaluable as the challenges of the disease become apparent.

10. Holidays

HOW CAN YOU make the holidays enjoyable and memorable?

Holidays often bring back wonderful memories of times when there was shared laughter, visits with family and friends, and past celebrations and traditions. You or your loved one with dementia may, at these special times, experience a longing for those past times as you cope with new and challenging situations.

Holiday celebrations can present new opportunities, too. Trying to maintain your traditional holiday events and family gatherings can lead to feelings of anxiety, loneliness, and frustration. Finding balance between those activities that are necessary and those that can be changed is the first step to recognizing what really is important in making the holidays meaningful. Caregivers must be realistic about the energy and time needed to continue the traditions that matter most to someone with Alzheimer's disease.

Ask others for help in implementing those traditions that you and the entire family think should be kept. Don't expect the person with dementia to participate to the extent that he did previously. Identify a "quiet" room if things get too hectic for the person with dementia, and have someone familiar stay with the person so that he does not feel isolated. Maintain a safe environment by avoiding confusing decorations, edible decorations, or cluttered walkways. Plan events and celebrations earlier in the day if the person with dementia has begun to show signs of agitation in the evening.

When choosing gifts for the person with Alzheimer's disease, it can be helpful to remember the following:

* Individuals in the Early-to-Mild stage often are aware of their limitations and need gifts and celebrations that

enhance their remaining abilities. These individuals often still have communication skills, can be active, and also want to maintain their independence. Good gifts are those that encourage pleasant memories, socialization, and activity.

* In the Moderate stage, individuals usually have difficulty with daily activities and also with communication and attention span. Gifts for these individuals need to foster the preservation of remaining skills. Activities and socialization are important. Gifts should simplify daily activities of dressing or grooming: for example, tube socks that cannot be put on the wrong way and other simple, manageable clothing. Music, tapes, videos, or photo albums of family gatherings can renew special memories. The person with Alzheimer's disease might enjoy a bird feeder and tape of bird songs. Filling the feeders and supplying the water is a way of showing care.

* In the Severe Stage, individuals usually have very short attention spans, impaired mobility, poor communication skills, and problems with complex tasks. Gifts at this stage should stimulate the senses and make the individual "feel good" if possible. Gifts that stimulate the sense of touch, such as a stuffed animal, pillow, or soft lap robes are very comforting and appropriate. Visual stimulation is possible with colorful mobiles and window prisms that capture sunlight. Music, especially that which has been pleasing for the person in the past or a tape of a loved one's voice, can be reassuring and soothing. A visit with a small pet can stimulate touch and bring back pleasant memories of childhood pets.

Address each holiday as a new adventure. Develop "new traditions" that incorporate your loved one's remaining skills.

11. Telling Young Children

HOW DO YOU tell young children that a family member has Alzheimer's disease?

If the relative with Alzheimer's disease lives with the family, the telling will be gradual. Young children most likely will notice that the person sits for long periods and often just rocks or sleeps in a chair. They may notice that the person has to be told to eat and, even may have to be helped to eat. They may notice that the person tries to assist in various activities, but can't seem to remember what to do or how to follow directions.

If the relative does not live with the family, and children see the loved one less frequently, they will notice a lapse in the person's memory or a change in behavior. They may become scared or wonder what's happening. Most children will find it difficult to comprehend why the person with Alzheimer's disease calls him or her by another name or unexpectedly asks, "Who are you?" When children notice these and other differences, it is time to straightforwardly tell them what is happening.

* Children need to know that the person has a disease that causes a loss of memory. More importantly, they need to know that, despite the memory loss, the person loves them as much as ever. The children need to know that if the relative becomes angry or agitated, it is because the person is feeling frustrated or helpless, not because she loves them any less.

* Children also need to be encouraged to spend time with the person with Alzheimer's disease, even when her memory fades so much that she no longer recognizes who she is conversing with.

* Tell your children that, as the disease progresses, they may have to help the loved one by reading to the person with dementia, telling stories, playing simple games, or helping them tie shoes or put on coats or sweaters.

Read to your children stories about other children who live with someone who has Alzheimer's disease. Four recommended readings are:

* *Remember Grandma?* **Laura Langston. Viking, 2004.** Grandma lives with Margaret's family. She and Marga-

ret go for walks, sing together, and gather apples to make Grandma's special mile-high apple pie. But more and more, Grandma can't remember the names of things. And, at one point, she doesn't even know Margaret. This hurts so much that Margaret goes to her room without giving Grandma a hug. Her Mom, in an attempt to console her, tells her that Grandma's brain is all mixed up, but that she still loves her even if she can't remember her name. Margaret gradually adjusts to what's happening in Grandma's brain and creatively continues to do loving things with her, even crawling into Grandma's lap and telling her, "I am Margaret, I am your remembering." This is a wonderful story that gently reassures readers about the love within families that endures even when memory does not.

* *Belle Teal.* **Ann M. Martin. Scholastic, 2001.** Belle Teal is a fifth grader who lives with her Mom and Gran way out in the country. Their life isn't easy but they get by. They don't have much money but Belle Teal feels rich with their love. The new school year presents many unexpected challenges. But an even bigger problem is that Gran's memory is slipping away. Her mama works longer hours to support the family, which means that Belle Teal and Gran have to find their way in doing the things that need to be done. With the problems both at school and at home, Belle Teal's world almost falls apart until she discovers the importance of sticking together—as a family, as a town, and as friends. This is an honest and moving story of a young girl and two strong women facing major challenges and succeeding.

* *What's Happening to Grandpa?* **Maria Shriver. Little, Brown & Co., 2004.** This story is about Katherine's experience with her Grandfather, who is beginning to repeat the same stories. He also keeps asking the same question, over and over, and can't seem to remember what he has just done. It frightens her when he yells at her grandmother, and it worries her when he doesn't remember her name. It's clear to her that something is

wrong and she asks her Mom, "What's happening to Grandpa?" Her Mom tells her that her Grandpa has Alzheimer's disease and explains some of what happens to a person who has the disease. Katherine is stunned and wonders what to do in the face of it all. Her mother looks her in the eyes and says, "Honey, what we do now is support Grandma and just keep on loving and respecting Grandpa the way we always have." Katherine resolves to cherish her Grandpa's life and memories. In creatively doing so, she forges a bond between them that will remain forever in their hearts. This story is not only about Katherine's grandpa; it's about the author's father.

* *Naming Maya.* **Uma Krishnaswami. Farrar Straus Giroux, 2004.** Maya, whose home is in New Jersey, is spending part of her summer in Chennai, India, with her mother, who is trying to sell Maya's grandfather's old house. While there, she learns much about her family's culture and history and much about the choosing of her name, which she believes may have contributed to her parent's divorce. However, the most intriguing part of the story happens as Maya is drawn into a complicated friendship with eccentric Kamala Mami, who has been a housekeeper and cook for years in Maya's extended family. Maya notices that Kamala Mami forgets things she promises to remember and begins to exhibit worrying behaviors. They make a pact that Maya will not tell her Mother or anyone else what is going on in Kamala Mami. Gradually, Maya cannot keep her part of the promise and Kamala Mami is hospitalized. One of the most exquisite parts of the story happens when Kamala Mami gives Maya a little accordion-folded book with parchment pages bent from age and use. The gift helps Maya understand where her name comes from. It is also a way for Kamala Mami to thank Maya for caring for her and protecting her when she was becoming more and more confused.

Most children take their cues from their parents. For children to adapt well and continue to show love and respect for the person with Alzheimer's disease, it is important that their parents model this kind of behavior. Amazingly, children adapt sometimes more easily than do adults. When the person with Alzheimer's disease does not remember, a child may promise to be his "rememberer." A child may more easily and readily hug the person or spend time just being near him. This is the type of unconditional love that speaks more clearly than words.

12. Spirituality

HOW ARE THE SPIRITUAL dimensions of persons with Alzheimer's disease and their caregivers, family members, and friends affected during the Alzheimer's disease process?

Concerning the person with Alzheimer's Disease:

* As many answers exist to the question concerning spiritual dimensions and Alzheimer's disease as there are persons who have had Alzheimer's disease. Each answer is different, because each person has her individual relationship with a Spiritual Being.

* Each of us is intrigued about our inner self. Self-reflection continues throughout the progression of Alzheimer's disease, so that the person's inner self is active. Caregivers, family members, and friends can assist the loved one by supporting the religious tradition that person followed all her life. If no formal religious tradition exists, family members, caregivers, and friends need to seek ways to help lift the spirits of the person. It may be walks outside enjoying nature, the cultivation of beautiful gardens, listening to favorite music, painting, or drawing.

* Along this spiritual journey pastors, priests, religious directors, rabbis, or other individuals can help. There will be times when loved ones express their concerns and grief. Statements like "I must have been very bad in my life to have God give me this," can be disturbing to caregivers, family members, and friends, but it is

important to help the person reflect on her grief with others. This is where spiritual leaders can be helpful.

* For those who have participated in organized religious traditions, caregivers, family members, and friends need to dialogue with the religious congregations about the person's spiritual needs, wants, and desires and about changes in health or living situations. Spiritual leaders of all faith traditions generally will help the loved one maintain her spiritual life. Hospice workers are specially trained to accommodate spiritual issues in end-of-life situations.

Concerning caregivers, family members, and friends:

* Those who have been caregivers for someone through the progressing stages of Alzheimer's disease will tell you that their own faith has been tested and grown.

* The process of grief and denial occurs throughout the progression of the disease, as the caregiver, family members, and friends witness the effects of the gradual deterioration.

* Caregivers, family members, and friends are tempted to talk about the loved one as if he or she were not there. By doing so the person with Alzheimer's disease loses dignity and is reduced to an object. Caregivers, family members, and friends should treat the person with Alzheimer's disease with the respect and dignity due another human being, recognizing preserved abilities and the person's spiritual dimension. This can be a challenge. It helps if you remember that the deterioration is not the fault of the loved one but is due to the disease.

* Grief is real for caregivers, family members, and friends. Questions arise such as: "How can this be happening to Mom? She doesn't deserve this," or "Why do I have to be the primary caregiver? I had other things planned for my life."

* Caregivers, family members, and friends need just as much spiritual support as do loved ones with the dis-

ease. They need compassion, not pity, from their own family members, colleagues at work, friends, and relatives. When the loved one slips into the stage where she is not as self-reflective, those living and working with the loved one retain memories of what life was like before the progression of the disease.

✳ Many bonds of friendship are formed as caregivers, family members, and friends go through the progression of Alzheimer's disease with loved ones. These bonds and times of extraordinary spiritual development are life-long gifts.

Grant that I may not criticize my neighbor until I have walked a mile in his moccasins.

—Native American Prayer

Resources Available for Those Affected with Alzheimer's Disease, Their Caregivers, Family Members, and Friends

Resources

Local Resources

AS OUR POPULATION grows older, people increasingly want to direct their own care. Many resources are available to help in making choices about living arrangements: in-home care, assisted-living facilities, nursing home, and rehabilitation centers.

Persons affected by Alzheimer's disease, their caregivers, family members, and friends all can be involved in choosing the best care that will carry out the wishes of the person with the disease. All involved in helping someone with suspected Alzheimer's disease should become familiar with the following resources:

* **Your Local Area Office on Aging and Local Alzheimer's Association Chapter.** Their numbers are listed in your phone directory. They have multiple resources and are connected with local and national networks to help all those living and working with Alzheimer's disease.

* **Geriatric Evaluation & Mental Health Programs.** The geriatric evaluation process works with patients and their families to provide comprehensive assessment and planning for ongoing care.

* **Geriatric Case/Care Management Services.** Geriatric case/care management is a professional service that provides a wide array of services for older adults. Most case managers provide a home assessment and then create a recommended care plan based on the inter-

view. The goal of the case manager is to set up services that allow for a safe environment for the senior living at home. Once living at home is no longer an option, the case manager can handle placement into another setting providing a higher level of care.

* **Home Health Companies.** Home health care companies include home health agencies, referral registries, and non-medical companion services. Home health care is, simply put, health care delivered in the patient's home. Services may range from at-home nursing care following a hospital stay to ongoing assistance with daily living activities such as bathing. Thanks to technological advances, many procedures that were previously performed in a medical facility now can be safely and efficiently administered in the home setting.

* **Living Options.** Living options include independent-living retirement communities, public-assisted housing for the elderly, assisted-living facilities, assisted-living facilities specializing in Alzheimer's disease and dementia, nursing homes, rehabilitation centers, and transitional care units. Find a local agency or nonprofit organization that has a listing of resources to help you decide what is appropriate care for your loved one.

* **Hospice Programs.** Hospice services are available to persons who no longer benefit from curative treatment. To receive hospice service, a person must be willing to serve as the patient's primary caregiver. The patient must be alert and understand the services that are to be provided. The physician normally refers the patient to the hospice program, and Medicare generally covers services.

Alzheimer's Disease Information on the Internet

THE FOLLOWING WEB sites are intended to provide you with health information. They are not substitutes for consultation with a health professional.

General Health Information on the Internet

* **MedlinePlus** (http://www.medlineplus.gov), a resource of the National Library of Medicine, is an easy-
  to-use, online web site that provides extensive information from the National Institutes of Health and other
  trusted sources on over 650 diseases and conditions.
  Along with the Health Topics section that links to over-
  views, treatment options, research, and more, lists of
  hospitals and physicians are presented as well. A medical encyclopedia and a medical dictionary, extensive
  information on prescription and nonprescription
  drugs, health information from the media, and links to
  thousands of clinical trials are also available.

* **The Medical Library Association (MLA)** produces a
  list of the "Top Ten Most Useful Web Sites" (http://
  www.mlanet.org/resources/medspeak/topten.html).
  The Consumer and Patient Health Information Section (CAPHIS) of MLA also has created "a Websites
  You Can Trust" page at http://caphis.mlanet.org/
  consumer/index.html.

Web Sites Devoted to Alzheimer's Disease

SEVERAL ORGANIZATIONS EXIST that focus on Alzheimer's Disease, and these organizations also provide web sites written
so that the general public can learn more about the disease.

* **Alzheimer's Disease Education & Referral Center
  (ADEAR)** (http://www.alzheimers.org/) is a service
  of the National Institute on Aging. It provides current
  up-to-date information on Alzheimer's disease for
  health care professionals, for people who suffer from
  Alzheimer's disease, and for their families, as well as
  for the general public. Sections include: A General
  Overview of Information on Alzheimer's, Caregiving,
  Health Information, Publications, and Resources.

* **Alzheimer's Association** (http://www.alz.org/) is a
  voluntary health organization that provides information and care consultation, funds for research, and

more. This web site provides resources that include health information in many languages, a section for Care Partners, advocacy, the latest in research, and more.

* **The Fisher Center for Alzheimer's Research Foundation** (http://www.alzinfo.org/) works to create an online community that includes the use of chat rooms, message boards, and a vast array of online databases of information on Alzheimer's Disease. Sections include: About Alzheimer's, Find Doctors and Other Services, Community, News, and Get Involved.

* **Alzheimer Research Forum** (http://www.alzforum. org/) is a nonprofit web site established to serve the scientific and clinical research community as well as the general public. The Disease Management section on the left hand side of the page is useful. A section on Caregiving is also presented.

* **NIHSeniorHealth.Gov** includes a section on "Alzheimer's Disease" (http://nihseniorhealth.gov/alzheim ersdisease/toc.html), with topics that include defining Alzheimer's, causes and risk factors, symptoms and diagnosis, treatments and research, and more. "Caring for Someone with Alzheimer's" (http://nihsenior health.gov/alzheimerscare/toc.html) includes sections on home care, residential care, safety issues, and caregiver support.

* **Alzheimer's Disease Page** (http://alzheimer.wustl. edu/adrc2/) is sponsored by the Washington University Alzheimer's Disease Research Center in St. Louis, Missouri. Some of the information on this page is specific to the St. Louis area, but general overview sections are also available on several topics.

Early-Onset Alzheimer's Disease

THE ALZHEIMER'S ASSOCIATION has produced a brochure on "Living With Early-Onset Alzheimer's Disease" (http://www. alz.org/Resources/FactSheets/Brochure_LivingwithEarlyOn setAD.pdf).

Web Sites for Specific Racial/Ethnic Groups

* **MedlinePlus** has a Spanish Language portal (http://medlineplus.gov/spanish/). The MedlinePlus Health Topics on Alzheimer's Disease and for Alzheimer's Caregivers both have a Spanish Language version that brings together resources that are available online in Spanish (http://www.nlm.nih.gov/medlineplus/spanish/alzheimersdisease.html and http://www.nlm.nih.gov/medlineplus/spanish/alzheimerscaregivers.html).

* **The Alzheimer's Association Diversity Toolbox** (http://www.alz.org/Resources/Diversity/overview.asp) includes resources for Black/African American, Chinese, Hispanic/Latino, and Korean communities. The toolbox also includes a link to language-specific materials for the groups highlighted. The Alzheimer's Association also has a Spanish Language gateway (http://www.alz.org/hispanic/overview_sp.asp).

* **The National Network of Libraries of Medicine** (NN/LM) "Multilingual Health Information" (http://nnlm.gov/train/chi/multi.html) lists numerous web sites that provide health information in languages other than English.

* For caregiver information in other languages, see the **Family Caregiver Alliance** web site (http://www.caregiver.org/caregiver/jsp/content_node.jsp?nodeid=834). Resources are currently available in Spanish and Chinese.

Web Sites Focusing on Issues Dealing with Senior Health Concerns

* **The National Institute on Aging** (http://www.nia.nih.gov/) is one of the National Institutes of Health, and it focuses on research on the aging process and issues related to age. In addition to research, the insti-

tute looks for ways to disseminate their findings to health care providers as well as the general public. They have partnered with the National Library of Medicine to create NIHSeniorHealth.Gov (http://nihsenior health.gov/). NIHSeniorHealth makes aging-related health information easily accessible for family members and friends seeking reliable, easy-to-understand online health information. The senior-friendly format allows for high contrast and large text, as well as including an audio button to have the text read aloud for the person with low vision or low literacy skills. Site also includes topics on Alzheimer's disease, arthritis, balance problems, caring for someone with Alzheimer's disease, hearing loss and more.

* **The United States Administration on Aging (AoA)** (http://www.aoa.gov) from the Department of Health and Human Services provides a general overview on issues related to aging. Click on Elders and Families to find the Alzheimer's Resource Room.

Many web sites include sections devoted to health concerns of senior citizens. MedlinePlus lists Senior Health Topics at http://www.nlm.nih.gov/medlineplus/seniorshealth.html. The CAPHIS web site You Can Trust includes a section on Senior Health Issues (http://caphis.mlanet.org/consumer/consumerSeniors.html).

Financial Help Programs

MANY PROGRAMS PROVIDE financial help for doctor's visits, prescriptions, and other types of assistance that the person with Alzheimer's disease might qualify for.

* **Benefits Check-Up** (http://www.benefitscheckup.org/) allows people over 55 years of age to locate programs that can assist them in paying for prescription drugs, health care, housing, utility costs and more.

* **Alzheimer's Association Resources on Financial Matters** (http://www.alz.org/People/Planning/

FinancialMatters.asp) provides links and information on health care insurance, personal resources, and Social Security.

* **The Fisher Center for Alzheimer's Research Foundation** "Paying For Healthcare" (http://www.alzinfo.org/resources/paying/default.aspx) gives ideas for understanding options and programs for paying for treatment costs.

* For resources in prescription drug programs, see Benefits Check-up. Also available are "Together Rx Access" (http://www.togetherrxaccess.com/) and "Rx Hope" (http://www.rxhope.com/).

* For a more complete list of programs, see the NN/LM MidContinental Region web site section on issues related to low-income health concerns at http://nnlm.gov/mcr/resources/community/inner.html This page includes a section on insurance and prescription drug resources.

Newsletters and E-mail Alerts

YOU CAN RECEIVE an alert when the ADEAR *Connections* newsletter or other ADEAR materials are published, including an Alzheimer's Disease Clinical Trials alert, and National Institute on Aging News Releases by subscribing at http://209.70.85.96/adearalert/lists/?p=subscribe&id=4.

* **The Alzheimer's Association** publishes Advances, a quarterly newspaper that is distributed through its chapters. You can see the online back issues for 1999–2003 at http://www.alz.org/Resources/Newsletters.asp.

* **The National Library of Medicine** issues e-mail news updates, and you can subscribe through MedlinePlus at http://www.nlm.nih.gov/cgi/medlineplus/listserv.pl?lang=EN. You can choose from general health news or from specialty topics, including senior health.

Research on Alzheimer's Disease

❋ **ADEAR** has developed a resource page that lists the many online resources you can use to research scientific databases (http://www.alzheimers.org/litsearchchid. htm).

❋ **The National Library of Medicine's** free online database PubMed (http://www.pubmed.gov) has over 15 million citations for biomedical articles dating back to the 1950s. PubMed includes links to many sites that provide full-text articles and other related resources. To help you, "preformulated" searches are available on MedlinePlus (http://medlineplus.gov). Each of the health topics includes a link in the left bar in the yellow box titled "Search MEDLINE/PubMed for recent research articles on." Clicking on this will automatically start a search for the latest research articles in PubMed on that topic.

Articles Written about Alzheimer's Disease

ONCE YOU GET CITATIONS for articles written about Alzheimer's disease, you can obtain the articles from many academic, hospital, and public libraries having consumer health collections. To locate the one nearest you, go to the library directory on MedlinePlus (http://www.nlm.nih.gov/medlineplus/ libraries.html). Many hospital and medical libraries also are open to the public for walk-in service. Although you cannot check out their materials, you are allowed access to journals and textbooks while in the library. Call your local hospital or university to find out their policy. Public libraries are always available to assist the public with their information needs.

Support Groups

❋ The AOA has compiled a state contact list of Family Caregiver Support Programs. It is available at http://

www.aoa.gov/prof/aoaprog/caregiver/careprof/
state_by_state/state_contact.asp.

* The Family Caregiver Alliance lists four online support
groups at http://www.caregiver.org/caregiver/jsp/
content_node.jsp?nodeid=347.

Hospice and Palliative Care

THE GREEN-FIELD RESOURCE CENTER staff have compiled a list of
resources on the Alzheimer's Association web site at http://
www.alz.org/Resources/Resources/rtrlhospice.asp. The library does not lend items from its collection directly to the
public; they do, however, lend items through local Alzheimer's
Association chapters. If you wish to borrow an item on this
list, you may do so through your local chapter or local library.

Spirituality

FOR MATERIALS ON THE specific topic of grief and bereavement
consult Green-Field Library's Hospice and Palliative Care in
Alzheimer's Disease resource list at http://www.alz.org/
Resources/Resources/rtrlhospice.asp.

Some recommended reading for caregivers and those with
Alzheimer's disease include:

* Iris, M. (1998) *Spiritual traditions and aging.* Park Ridge
Center Bulletin 6:12 Park Ridge, IL: Park Ridge Center
for Health, Faith, and Ethics. Seven issues emerge from
a study on how older people experience the religious
and spiritual aspects of life. http://www.parkridge
center.org/Page109.html.

* Post, S.G. *God and Alzheimer's: a neurological reflection
on religious experience, self, and soul.* Park Ridge Center
Bulletin 19:9–10. Park Ridge, IL: Park Ridge Center
for Health, Faith, and Ethics. An online article on the
relationship between personhood, self-identity, and

God in persons with Alzheimer's disease. http://
www.parkridgecenter.org/Page482.html.

* Alternative Solutions. *Alternative solutions in long-term
care—spirituality.* Sparta, NJ: Alternative Solutions. A
comprehensive collection of spirituality links to organizations providing resources and services for health care
professionals and caregivers, recreation therapists, activity directors, social workers, and creative arts spe-
cialists. http://www.activitytherapy.com/spirit.htm.

* Mayo Clinic. *Spirituality and Alzheimer's disease.* Roches-
ter, MN: Mayo Clinic. A web page highlighting the
significance of rituals, caring for the caregiver, and the
forms of spirituality. http://www.mayoclinic.com/
invoke.cfm?objectid=8E184EA1-D0C2-459A-
891CE75B96C2D3DD.

* Post, S.G. Alzheimer's & grace. *First Things* April 2004;
vol. 142, pp. 12–14. http://www.firstthings.com/
ftissues/ft0404/opinion/post.html.

Other sources for information on spirituality and caregiving include:

* The Center for Aging, Religion, and Spirituality, in St.
Paul, Minnesota, provides educational programming,
conducts research, and produces publications that ex-
plore the relationship between aging and spirituality.
Their web site is accessible at http://www.aging-
religion-spirituality.com.

* Outreach to Faith Communities Kit. Kensington, MD:
National Family Caregiver's Association. Three down-
loadable faith services (Interfaith, Lutheran, and Catho-
lic) to use for worship with caregivers. Follow the How-
to Guides link on the home page. http://www.
nfcacares.org.

*I expect to pass through this world but once. Any good
therefore that I can do or any kindness that I can show for
fellow creature, let me do it now. Let me not defer or neglect
it, for I shall not pass this way again.*
—Stephen Grellet (1773–1855), a French-born Quaker

Index

National Institute on Aging,
105–106
National Institute on Aging
News Releases, 107
National Library of Medicine,
106–107
free online database, PubMed,
108
resource of, 103
National Network of Libraries of
Medicine, 105
Newsletters, 107
NIHSeniorHealth.gov, 104, 106
NN/LM MidContinental Region
web site, 107
Nonverbal cues, 63
Normal changes of aging, demen-
tia, distinguishing, 8–11
Nursing home care, 102
cost, 76

Office on Aging, 101
Other illnesses, 79–80
Other person's point of view, 6
Outreach to Faith Communities
Kit, 110
Overmedication, 79

Pacing, 61
Palliative care, 109
Patience, importance of, 49–50
Patient's bill of rights, 18, 20
Personal hygiene, 7
Pet therapy programs, 8, 57
Pneumonia, gastrointestinal
infection, 80
Positive environment, creation of,
47–49
Positive outlook, 6
Power of attorney, 78–79
Pre-Alzheimer's stage, 3–20
brain functions in, 4–8, 12–16
ambulation, 7
complex tasks, 6
early-to-mild stage, 14
judgment/reasoning, 7

language, 5
memory, 5
moderate stage, 14–15
senses, 8
severe stage, 15–16
social skills, 6–7
caregiver's perspective, 16–18
early-to-mid stage, 16–17
moderate stage, 17
severe stage, 17–18
definition of Alzheimer's
disease, 11–12
life-altering experience, Alzheimer's disease as, 18–19
normal changes of aging, dementia, distinguishing,
8–11
overview, 3–5
patient's bill of rights, 18, 20
scenario, 3
Prescription drug programs, 107
Preserved skills timeline, 13
Pressure sores, 67
Privacy, 85
Progression of Alzheimer's disease in brain, 12–16. *See
also* Brain changes; Function of brain
early-to-mild stage, 14
moderate stage, 14–15
severe stage, 15–16
Psycho-motor functioning, 9
Public-assisted housing, 102

Racial/ethnic groups, web sites
for, 105
Recognition, 61
Referral registries, 102
Rehabilitation centers, 102
Remember Grandma? Langston,
Laura, 92–93
Research on Alzheimer's disease,
108
Resources, 100–110
Respect, importance of, 18
Rhythm, 86
"Rx Hope," 107